A Piece of Her Mind

Mike & Kris —
Thank you for your
support & encouragement.
Enjoy our book :)
Mona

DREAM BIG
& Stacy

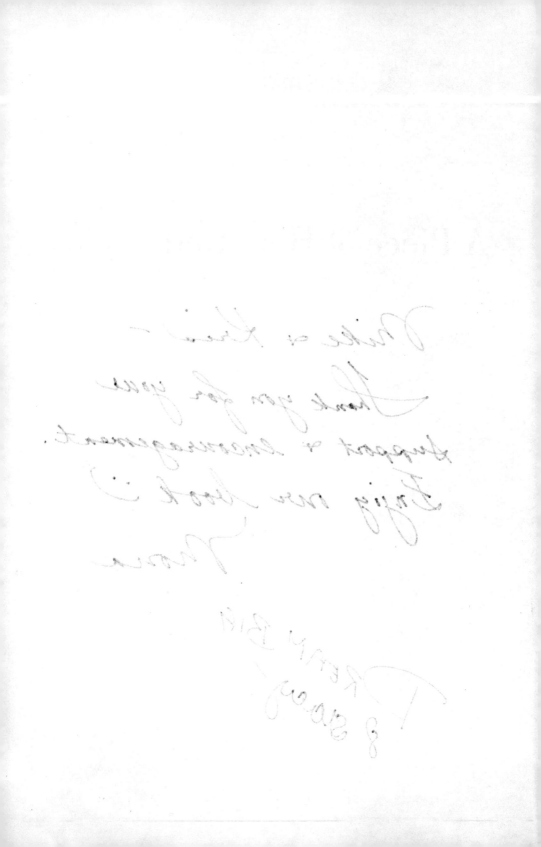

A Piece of Her Mind

A Mother-Daughter Journey
Through Stroke and Recovery

Mona Gupton & Stacy Gupton

To order additional copies of this book, contact:
Xlibris Corporation
1-888-795-4274
www.Xlibris.com
Orders@Xlibris.com
64569

Contents

DEDICATION

*I think a hero is an ordinary individual who
finds strength to persevere and endure
in spite of overwhelming obstacles.*

~Christopher Reeves~

This book is dedicated to stroke survivors everywhere, and in particular, my daughter Stacy. I am astounded by her strength, perseverance, and determination to defy the odds. She is truly remarkable. The wit and humor she exhibits everyday have helped me lean toward the acceptance she had no choice in. I have no doubt she will leave an indelible mark on the world and make it a better place. She is my hero.

Introduction

Six and a half years ago, in April of 2003, my family and I were introduced to stroke on a very personal level when my youngest daughter Stacy suffered a massive stroke at age twenty-one. Since then the occurrence of stroke in the United States has risen to one every forty seconds. Stroke statistics are absolutely frightening. According to the American Heart Association and the Centers for Disease Control and Prevention in *Heart Disease and Stroke Statistics—2009 Update*, approximately 795,000 Americans suffer a stroke over the course of a year. Stroke results in more serious long-term disabilities than any other disease. Worldwide the number of people suffering a stroke is a staggering 15 million annually.

The report contains more alarming data. Stroke is the third leading cause of death in this country. In 2005, it accounted for one in 17 deaths in the United States. More women than men die from stroke. The death rate for women from stroke is twice that of breast cancer. When they survive stroke, women tend to have higher degrees of disability and more difficulty doing routine activities afterward.

Stroke statistics are largely ignored because stroke is generally thought of as an older person's health issue. The National Stroke Association reports that one in three Americans cannot name a single stroke symptom. Because most of us do not recognize the symptoms, we fail to treat stroke as the life-threatening emergency it is. The majority of people, if asked, would not know that stroke can happen to anyone, at any age, anywhere, anytime.

Four out of five American families will be impacted by stroke in the near future if the statistics stay where they are. Our decision to share our story, Stacy's story, came from our desire to make others aware of what stroke is and what it does. We entered into our relationship with stroke ignorant and vulnerable, so we hope to spare others the same fate. We feel strongly that by sharing what happened to Stacy we can help someone else who has suffered from a stroke, traumatic illness, or life-altering injury. Ultimately we want to see the numbers go down. We cannot stress strongly enough the need for advocacy on the part of stroke survivors. Most important is our goal of facilitating awareness. Though the actual stroke happens only to the victim, it impacts every member of that person's family. Surviving stroke requires a team effort and a resolve to never give up.

Please join me as my family and I share an adventure, a soul-searching marathon, a spiritual and emotional weathering, and an arrival at a destination I wondered if we could ever reach: acceptance. If you take nothing more from this story, remember this: If stroke happens every forty seconds, eventually you or someone close to you will experience its devastation. Recognize the symptoms. Obtain immediate medical attention for anyone who experiences sudden numbness on one side of the body, sudden confusion, problems seeing, standing, walking, or speaking, or sudden severe headache that comes out of nowhere. Not all of these symptoms occur with every stroke so do not ignore any of them even if they improve. Know what to do if stroke does strike. If you suspect stroke or if the person in question exhibits any of the symptoms listed, follow these steps. First, ask the person to smile. Does one side of their face droop? Ask the person to raise both arms. Does one arm drop? Ask the person to repeat a simple sentence. Are their words slurred? Did he or she repeat the sentence? If you, your friend, family member or even a stranger exhibits any of these symptoms, remember time is precious. Call 911—get help. By doing so you could save a life, perhaps even your own.

Chapter One

Road Trip

A journey of a thousand miles begins with a single step.

~Lao-tzu~

The majority of books I've read about overcoming personal tragedy describe the event and the aftermath as a journey. When we decided to write about Stacy's stroke I tried to find a different analogy—something new to entice the reader. I struggled for months but kept coming back to the emotional rollercoaster ride—the peaks and valleys—of the early minutes and hours. Every day brought unexpected twists or turns. Finally I concluded that a journey was exactly what our story entailed. I could find no better slant for telling someone about what happened to Stacy and our family. Once I made that decision I moved forward with a question.

How do you adequately describe a journey? What word or words should you use? You could call it a jaunt; a trip, or a trek. Travel or passage may be the right word. A junket, a pilgrimage, or an odyssey might be your choice. Regardless of the word used to tell someone about leaving one place and arriving in another, the idea behind that concept is that of being prepared for the event that is about to take place. If you know you are leaving home, you pack a toothbrush, a change of clothes, clean underwear, and other essentials. You fill your car with gas. You make sure you have some money and your passport. There is a sense of anticipation in knowing, even partially, where you intend to end up.

I am a planner and a logical person. I like to know where I need to be and what I need to do. If I know what's expected of me I will do it to the best of my ability. I can improvise when necessary but I prefer being prepared. I don't like guess work and hate to be late. If I know I'm going on vacation on Tuesday, my bag is packed the week before. The essential ingredients for my Thanksgiving dinner are in my pantry, freezer, and refrigerator at least two weeks before the holiday. I have my Christmas shopping done weeks if not months in advance. I am not a fly-by-the-seat-of-my-pants kind of person. I detest being caught off guard. At one point in my life I was of the opinion that nothing should come as a surprise if you are in tune with your environment. I do not feel that way any longer. Experiences over the past six years have taught me otherwise.

Some of the excursions we take in life catch us totally unprepared although each of us knows that life can irrevocably transform in an instant. We all know nothing can remain unchanged yet sometimes we find ourselves in a situation where what we knew or thought we knew suddenly escapes our realm of thinking and is replaced by uncertainly. We ask ourselves, "How did that happen? How did I get here from there?" We search but cannot find an answer that makes sense.

My faith in God has always sustained me. I trust that everything happens for a reason, yet prior to this experience there was a part of me that insisted there should be an unmistakable warning of some kind when one was about to experience a life-altering event. You know, like a loud bell or bright flashing light. A signal so obvious no one could ignore it. Big bold letters with the words WATCH YOUR STEP! PROCEED WITH CAUTION! REDUCE SPEED! WARNING! WARNING! WARNING!

While I told myself then that my idea was really not an unreasonable expectation, I now know that if people actually had the power to foresee impending tragedy, to know what lies around the bend, few of us would have the courage to venture ahead knowing what was about to happen. My family has been 'on the road' so to speak for nearly seven years. The first leg of our journey was a bumpy ride indeed. Around each curve was an obstacle to maneuver over, under, or through. Mountains appeared, out of nowhere. We had to calculate each step of slippery uphill slopes. Intersections required thoughtful decision before we could proceed. Sometimes we'd move forward at a snail's pace. Next we'd take three steps backward. We sometimes had to retrace our steps and start over in another direction. Other times we would come to a complete stop, unable to move, or speed downhill out of control at ninety-miles-an-hour.

This experience has taught us painful, though tender and priceless, life lessons. Roll with the punches, expect the unexpected, hold tight to your faith, never say never, and appreciate each step you take. Today my family and I take nothing for granted. We find joy in knowing every day holds something to be thankful for—if it's only the fact that the sun rises that morning. To fully appreciate the value of this amazing place we are now, you need to know where we came from and what brought us here.

Chapter Two

Home is Where Your Story Begins

Be it ever so humble, there's no place like home.

~John Howard Payne~

I once read that there's no way to be a perfect mother and a million ways to be a good one. I was fortunate to have a mother that fell into the latter category although she's incredibly close to flawless in the eyes of her family. A woman clothed in strength and dignity like the one in Proverbs 31, my mother's entire life has revolved around her family. Another statement that comes to mind is the one that says the greatest gift a man can give his children is to love their mother. I wish I had written those two statements because they describe my parents, Jack and Dorothy Cooper, to a tee.

My siblings and I grew up in a home with little money but plenty of love. We never doubted that our parents cared for each of the eleven of us (yes, eleven!) as well as each other. Home was on the range—literally. Prior to retirement, my father was a hard working cowboy—the genuine article. Since then he has kept busy in a lucrative home-based business making equipment such as saddles, bridles, chaps, and reins for other working cowboys. My mother has always been a stay-at-home housewife. Together they are quite a team.

Generations of remarkable women on both sides of my family paved the way for their modern descendants. My paternal grandmother, Hattie Smith Cooper, was 102 years old when she passed. Born in 1896, she led a fascinating life on the remote plains of Nebraska and South Dakota. During her lifetime she saw her world evolve from horse and buggy to man on the moon. Her mother, Maud McKee Smith, was a nurse, a mid-wife really, and often had to leave home on a moment's notice to deliver babies or help the doctor with whatever he needed. Hattie, the oldest daughter, stayed at home with her younger siblings. She recalled managing the house—cooking, cleaning, and childcare—at age seven.

My maternal grandmother, Bernice Snyder Jensen, fought spinal cancer and the loss of her mobility in the 1930's when my mother was still a teenager. Determined to keep moving, she walked through her home, pushing a wooden chair in front of her. Cancer was a formidable foe but giving up was not part of her plan. That home was a log cabin built by her mother, Clara Wilson Snyder on a 160-acre homestead in South Dakota. Clara was a young widow with two small children to raise. She built a successful ranch by herself at a time when women typically had to have a husband in the picture to make that happen. Although the cabin no longer stands, the land she tended remains in the family to this day.

The strength and perseverance of these women and numerous others on our family tree runs through the veins of their daughters, granddaughters and each new generation of women born into our big wonderful family. Motherhood has been a cherished part of our legacy. Being a mother is an esteemed profession. My mother taught by example and instructed well. My siblings and I learned early how to work hard regardless of the task, pitch in wherever we were needed, do without when need be, and appreciate the little things.

Motherhood found me early in life although my parents would have preferred I waited. In 1974, at the age of 16, I quit high school and married a cowboy. Neil Gupton was my high school sweetheart. Together we had four daughters. Like my mother, I wanted nothing more than to be a good wife and mother. It was a much bigger task than I could have ever imagined. Neil's and my relationship was turbulent, often violent. Raising children while married to an abusive alcoholic man took a huge toll on me. Neil and I divorced in 1992. I was a shadow of my former self but fully committed to making my kids' future brighter than their past.

In 2003—thirty years into motherhood—I was a divorced woman in my forties. I am totally honest when I say I had few problems with my children even in their teenage years. They had their fair share of broken hearts, a couple of fender benders, a few too many beers on occasion, several heated arguments, numerous bad hair experiences, countless slammed doors, at least one broken window, plenty of late night whispered conversations, and thankfully no arrests.

I was lucky to have great kids. Each of my girls graduated from high school and entered college. My oldest daughter, Camy, made the decision to leave college after two years to get married. The marriage did not last but Camy survived her own divorce with unbelievable grace and was successfully raising her eight-year-old daughter, Jordyn, on her own. Adorably precocious, Jordyn was the apple of my eye. We shared a special connection. What I enjoyed most about grandparenthood was the lack of pressure to be perfect. I could go with the flow and be just fine. I felt so fortunate to have Camy and Jordyn nearby.

Patty, my second, was a kindergarten teacher in Houston—a long way from home she was thriving in the career she had chosen when she was in second grade. She had graduated college with a dual degree in elementary and early childhood education. Teaching children to read and write was as natural to her as breathing and she was a great teacher. She was in a serious relationship with a young man she met though mutual friends.

Third in line was Jeannie. Driven to succeed from an early age, she often pushed herself hard. Ever since her sophomore year of high school she had worked at least one job while carrying a heavy course load. She also lived in Houston, having relocated after college to work in retail management for a large home furnishings company. She had settled into life in a big city and shared an apartment with Patty. I was glad they had each other especially when holidays rolled around and they couldn't come home.

The baby of the group, Stacy, was a 21-year-old college junior. Majoring in art education she had plans to teach in an elementary setting like her sister. Parents of art students can sympathize with one another. My house and garage were full of projects in various degrees of completion. Sculptures, paintings and miscellaneous objects-de-art were in every corner and on every wall. Easels stood in the living room, spare bedroom and Stacy's own room as if they were part of the decor. The odor of turpentine was as common as the smell of chocolate chip cookies. Paintbrushes could be found soaking in my kitchen sink. Bits of wire, string, nuts and bolts, and anything Stacy found interesting had overtaken every plastic storage container in the house. Such is life with an artist.

Our lifestyle was a simple one with my meager income stretched to the limit. Each day brought a trial of one kind or other but we kept forging ahead. When we were knocked down, we got up. Life was not easy, but we were making it work. That became my philosophy, my mantra. "We will make it work; somehow; some way. Everything will work out in the end." We didn't have much in the way of money or material things but then who needs that stuff when you have each other?

Laramie, Wyoming—population 25,000 and elevation 7,200 feet—is a typical small town in the western United States. Home to the University of Wyoming where I have worked as an administrative assistant for almost eighteen years, Laramie has been home to us since 1985. The area holds so many memories. We came here as a family and stayed because Laramie had become our home.

At this point in our lives, finally free of fear, domination, and control, each of us was forging a path toward the future, together and separately. My girls had grown into remarkable young women. I was so proud of them. The four of them had a strong bond sharing victory and sorrow as only sisters can. On July 1, 2000—a few weeks before Stacy entered college—they officially sealed that bond with identical tattoos on the tops of their left feet—a four-part intertwined Celtic knot to represent their sisterhood. They designated that day their own special holiday—Sister Day.

April 2003—spring time in Wyoming. The landscape is grey on these windblown high plains. Winter is lengthy and keeps its icy grip on the countryside for months. That year we were all anxious to see the cold snowy season end. It had been a particularly long one or maybe it was just that it was a period of time that brought unexpected changes to our lives. We all had remarked on a number of occasions that it had already been a weird year.

The girls and I had all been together for Christmas but the holiday had been overshadowed by a visit to their terminally ill paternal grandfather, Chester Gupton. We drove north across Wyoming from Laramie to Sheridan together and visited the grandfather they hadn't seen in years. He had been a prominent figure in the girls' early childhood but after our divorce they had seen him only a couple of times and the interactions had been strained. As happens often in families, divorce influences the relationships children have with their grandparents and they are sometimes penalized for their parents' mistakes. Now cancer was ravaging Chet's body and his emotions were raw. He openly wept and was genuinely happy to see his granddaughters and me.

A bitter twist to Chet's final days was that Neil—his son, my ex-husband, the girls' dad—was in jail again on drunken driving charges and would have to remain there for at least six more months. The girls and I had been estranged from Neil for a number of years. His lifestyle and bad choices made it impossible for the girls to maintain any kind of association with him. During our visit with Chet we avoided the subject of Neil and kept the conversation light but as we were leaving my former father-in-law took my hand in his and said the only encouraging words he had ever spoken to me. "Mona, you did a hell of a job raising those girls by yourself." I thanked him and let him know how much his words meant to me. Prior to that conversation he had never acknowledged his son's shortcomings. There was a lot that went unsaid in that exchange but his meaning was clear to me.

When we celebrated Christmas a few days before our visit to their grandfather, Jeannie gifted Stacy with a journal—a beautiful book bound in green fabric with a colorful sequined design. On January 3, Stacy made an entry that would unknowingly define her year and her future.

> *Wow, it's 2003! It seems like just yesterday I was in high school, but I'm almost done with college. That scares me. I hope I can do it. Well, I thought I should write in this journal Jeannie gave me.*

I really don't know what to write, but I'm sure it will come to me. I can't stop thinking about Grandpa. Why do people have to die? I wish no one had to go through the pain. It kills me to think he could die any day and I might not have the chance to really get to know him. After everything that has happened in the last few months, I have thought a lot about life and how wonderful it is and how fast it can be taken from you. I think this year I will tell my friends and family how much they mean to me and not be afraid to let people into my life. I need to love myself and take care of myself so I can be a healthy person inside and out. That sounds corny but I really think I need that. Let the bad roll off and embrace the good in my life, and treat each day as my last and never look back on the bad stuff that has or might happen.

All of the girls wrestled with their grandfather's eminent death. However, it was Stacy who put her feelings on paper. Her journal entries in January revealed the sadness she was feeling for the man she wished she had known better.

I'm scared of death yet I know it will take his pain away. Is he in pain? That is something I need to know. Why do good people have to have so much pain in their lives? Does God really care about all of us? All I know is death scares me. I guess it's hanging over me, waiting to come down and take Grandpa Chet away from me. But He won't take everything from me! I will make it through this. I know I will!

A man of few words, Chet succumbed to his disease on February 8. The weather was horrible and Jordyn had the flu. Blowing snow and black ice forced road closures across the state. We did not make it to his funeral.

A few weeks later in mid-March, Camy, Jordyn, Stacy and I drove to Houston over Spring Break to spend time with Patty and Jeannie. We felt the need to regroup on a happier note. We enjoyed a week of warmth and sunshine. I visited Patty's kindergarten classroom and read books to her students. I had a delectable one-on-one lunch date with Jeannie at a seafood restaurant. We returned home to the aftermath of a vicious spring blizzard that had dropped nearly three feet of snow on Laramie and other parts of southeast Wyoming and northern Colorado. Our house and driveway were buried. We had to shovel snow before we could unpack from our trip. It took hours. The snow melted quickly. Subtle hints of spring could be seen if you searched for them—a few green blades of grass were dotting the yard. Warmer weather was on its way and the weird season would, with any luck, come to an end. Whew! It was all I could do not to sigh with relief.

Stacy was still living at home with me. It was easier and less expensive than living in the dorm or renting an apartment. She remarked often that she had the best roommate anyone could want. Her house buddy (me!) cooked and did laundry. The tiny rental house we had lived in since the divorce was finally less crowded. Stacy had been talking about possibly moving into her own place that coming summer but hadn't finalized any plans. We enjoyed an easy co-existence.

That Monday, April 10, began like a hundred other days. I rose at 6, made coffee and took a shower. Stacy had a routine of sleeping until the last second, jumping out of bed, throwing on a ball cap, and riding her bike or driving her Jeep to class. Today would be like that. I stuck my head in her doorway and said goodbye as I left for work. She mumbled in her sleep. I smiled to myself as I left. She had class at 9:00 in my building and then a break during which she would work a shift at the campus bookstore. She stopped briefly to borrow money for a Mountain Dew and then ran down the stairs with a quick goodbye. "See you later, Mom. Love you." Her last class of the day was one of her studio art classes. I expected her home about 7:00 for dinner. My expectation of an ordinary ending to this ordinary day would be shattered into a million tiny pieces. Life as we knew it was about to plunge off a cliff.

Chapter 3

A Bump in the Road

Courage is fear that has said its prayers.

~Dorothy Bernard~

Stacy arrived home later than usual that April night. She had stayed in the art studio to finish a class project. It was after 8:00 when she walked through the door and she was starving. She hurried through a meal of chicken enchiladas and began working on a different class assignment. This one was something! The students in the class were required to obtain objects from a flea market and transform them into something new. Stacy selected an old rotating television stand and a toilet seat. She used the items to create a one-of-a-kind swivel chair painted black and red that she fondly called "The Hot Seat."

It was so like Stacy to blend humor into a task. Her talent as an artist was emerging and it was fun to watch. Although she experimented with a variety of mediums, her painting preference, her passion, was oil or acrylic landscapes. Lately though, she had created a few dramatic abstract pieces that were really good.

Stacy's fifteen-credit-hour spring semester had been a bit challenging. Two of her five courses were studio classes that required a lot of extra time and effort but she didn't mind. She would have lived in the art studio if she could have. Two others were electives that she was enjoying immensely. The fifth was an art history class that was kicking her butt. She was having some trouble communicating with the professor and fully comprehending the expectations of the course. I quizzed her for hours on dates, artists, time periods, genres, and mediums. She told me many times that her head ached from the study exercises and exams. We both laughed at her valiant declaration, "I will pass this damn course or die trying!"

Stacy grabbed her tools and proceeded to finish assembling the chair. The colorful creation had occupied the center of my small living room for a couple of weeks and I had to admit, I was not going to be sad to see it go. I was as anxious for completion of this project as Stacy was! She knelt on the floor and began screwing the pieces together with a small cordless screwdriver. I was nearby cleaning up the dishes from dinner. Kneeling on all fours with her head tilted sideways, Stacy suddenly dropped the screwdriver, grabbed her head, and slumped to the floor. She groaned, "Oh, my head! Oh, God, it hurts! Oh, Mom, my head hurts."

For a brief second I thought she was joking. She had often remarked that she simply could not learn one more fact because her brain was full. It took only an instant to realize something was desperately wrong.

I rushed to Stacy's side. She crumpled forward in a heap—her body at an odd angle. When I tried to roll her over, she moaned and chanted, "It hurts! It hurts! It hurts!" Five feet five and one hundred twenty-five pounds, her small body was dead weight. Moving her took more strength than I expected. I finally was able to roll her onto her back. I was shocked to see her eyes—pupils huge, fixed and dilated. The left side of her face drooped. She drooled. Her voice sounded strange—her speech garbled. I know I stared at her because I was shocked by what I saw. My mind was racing. Silently, I screamed. *She's having a stroke. Oh, my God. She's having a stroke!*

I raced for the cordless phone, knelt again by Stacy's side and dialed 911. My heart pounded in my chest. My own voice sounded eerie, like it echoed in a barrel. "Please send an ambulance. My daughter collapsed. I think she's having a stroke." The dispatcher stayed on the line with me. I could hear the siren getting closer and closer. I ran to open the door. A police officer and three paramedics rushed in. The officer, a woman, told me I could hang up the phone. She asked me questions as the paramedics assessed Stacy. They loaded her onto the gurney and prepared to leave our house. I called Camy to tell her what happened and asked her to call her sisters in Texas. I grabbed my car keys, a jacket, and my purse and ran after the emergency personnel.

Laramie is such a small town; you can easily get from one side to the other in about ten minutes. The hospital is centrally located. As the ambulance pulled away from my driveway, I jumped into my car and drove to the emergency room. In route, the ambulance turned onto a different street so I actually arrived at the hospital before they did.

Emergency rooms exude fear and panic in my opinion. Regardless of how they are arranged, nothing can make them truly comfortable or inviting. That is not their intended purpose, after all. I rushed through the sliding doors with enough force to knock a moving freight train from its tracks. The first cubicle was empty and dark. On its door was a sign with a hand pointing to the next station. I ran toward it and spotted another sign that indicated I needed to wait until I was summoned. No one was ahead of me so I didn't wait.

Hospital admission paperwork can test the best of us. The female employee said, "Please be seated," and casually began gathering forms that she laid out in front of her. Generally calm in most situations, I momentarily fought the urge to rip this woman's arms off and beat her with them. I know she was trying to put me at ease but it wasn't working. I was as close to panic as I have ever been. Could she not see my anxiety? At one point I considered pushing her from her chair and taking over the data entry. Time seemed to be in some sort of strange suspended animation. Paperwork completed—I pushed through another door into the internal ER hallway.

As I ran down the hall the paramedics wheeled Stacy into an examination room. I was surprised and very relieved to see she was showing some slight improvement. Although she still wasn't moving normally and her speech was slurred, she smiled a lopsided grin at one of the paramedics and teased him a bit for not running the siren on the way to the hospital. I had been so overwhelmed by the situation I hadn't noticed that little detail. The paramedic explained that when a patient complains of severe headache, they typically do not run the siren. The young men gathered around Stacy's bed, teased her about her chair project, wished her well, and left the room. Nurses came in for their initial examination, completed the IV started in the ambulance, and summoned the on-call ER physician. It was approximately 9:00 p.m.

I stated my concern and my first thoughts to everyone I spoke to. I must have repeated myself a hundred times. "I think she had a stroke." Stacy couldn't bear to have the lights on so they kept the room as dark as possible. Suddenly and violently she vomited. I helped the nurse take her clothes off and put her into a gown. Her lifeless left side made the task difficult.

It was shortly after 10:00 p.m. when the doctor arrived. When he entered the room, he brushed past me and looked at Stacy's chart. Without waiting for him to ask, I rapidly gave him the details and finished with, "I think she is having a stroke." He asked me about medications she was taking. I stated, "None." He asked about her habits. I answered, "No smoking, very little drinking, decent diet, and regular exercise." I answered each of his questions as thoroughly as possible.

The doctor went on to ask for family medical history. One topic that caught his attention was the fact that I, and several other people in my family, had migraines on occasion. It had been years since I'd had one. I emphasized that Stacy had never had one. He returned to the subject of medications. Again I insisted that she took nothing. I repeated, "I think she had a stroke."

Dismissing my words, the doctor moved closer to me and asked about possible drug use. I insisted that Stacy did not use any drugs and rarely drank alcohol. He reached out and roughly grabbed my forearm. I was taken aback, stunned by his forceful words. "You might as well tell me what's she's on, because I'm going to find out anyway!" I was so shocked by his actions that my mouth dropped open. How absurd! It was ludicrous to think Stacy was on drugs. Pulling free, I firmly insisted that Stacy wasn't using anything. He muttered something about parents always being the last to know. In retrospect, I am certain that emergency room personnel, especially in a college town like Laramie, see evidence of every possible bad choice of the young adults who end up there. I swallowed my retort and tried to concentrate on Stacy.

The doctor continued his examination. He lifted Stacy's left hand. It plopped back onto the bed. His pen light caused her to wince when he checked her eyes. He asked her to smile. It was a crooked smile with only the right side of her mouth turning up. When she told him the right side of her neck hurt, her voice sounded thick like her tongue was swollen. He didn't respond. I asked him about a MRI. He abruptly said no, it was not necessary, but he would order a CT scan. He ordered some medication for pain and nausea.

I walked beside the gurney that carried Stacy down the sterile hallway to Radiology and waited while the CT scan was performed. Leaning my head against the wall while I stood outside the room, I tried to collect my thoughts and calm my fear. My heart still felt as if it would leap from my chest. I was terrified. I could not even imagine what Stacy was feeling. I kept thinking over and over. *What in the world is happening to her?*

Stacy was returned to the dark exam room where we waited. She was in agony and could not control the vomiting. It seemed to take forever for the doctor to return. He told us the CT scan revealed nothing conclusive. He performed a lumbar puncture, otherwise known as a spinal tap. Stacy cried through the painful procedure, holding my hand tightly in hers. When the doctor finished, he left the room and we waited for an answer. Again he informed us that the test had revealed nothing abnormal.

While we were waiting, Stacy's left side began to gradually regain function but her headache pain and nausea were still intense. She began vomiting again so more medication was administered. The doctor came back and gave us of his diagnosis—hemiplegic migraine—a rare headache that causes temporary paralysis. Bewildered, I wanted to hear more. I told the doctor I had never heard of this type of migraine. I went on to say no one I knew had ever experienced anything like that. Perhaps sensing my disbelief, he brusquely recommended working with our family physician to arrange a consultation with a neurologist. Laramie had none—we would need to leave town for a consult.

All I could do was hold the basin while Stacy vomited and wipe her mouth when she finished. The ER doctor admitted her to the hospital for overnight observation. It was already 5:00 a.m. when we moved into a regular hospital room. Stacy finally slept and I dozed in a nearby chair. My plan was to call our family doctor as soon as her office opened.

The sounds of an awakening town filtered through the windows shortly after we settled. One of the nurses came in and asked if I needed anything. She mentioned a fresh pot of coffee so I accepted a cup. I just sat and watched Stacy sleeping in the bed. At least she was peaceful now. Patty and Jeannie each called my cell phone on their way to work. An hour ahead, they wanted to know Stacy's status before they got busy with their day. Around 7:00 a.m. I quickly called Camy. I wanted to touch base with her before she and Jordyn left for school and work. I called my office to tell my co-workers where I was. Tracy Bennett, the department accountant took my call. My right hand at the office and a very good friend, Tracy told me not to worry about work. She insisted everyone would agree I was where I needed to be.

I watched the clock—silently willing the minutes to pass. I called the bookstore where Stacy worked and told her supervisor she would not be in. I called the Office of Student Life to request an excused absence from classes. When 8:30 finally came, I called our family doctor's office. We had been treated by a young local female physician for about four years. Stacy was rarely sick and had seen our doctor only a few times, the most recent for a cold before our trip to Texas. The doctor was already at the hospital for morning rounds so I expected her to stop by but she didn't. I called her office again around 9:30 and was told she would return to the hospital for rounds as soon as she had completed the day's appointments. Disappointed, I waited.

Stacy slept all day. Nurses came and went, checking her vital signs. Late in the afternoon she woke up and was able to move her left side again. I cannot describe how relieved I was to see that. A nurse and I helped her sit up. After several minutes on the edge of the bed, she made it to the bathroom with minimal assistance. Afterward, she crawled into the bed and slept again.

Early evening came and a nurse brought a dinner tray but Stacy didn't eat much. I nibbled, realizing it had been almost twenty-four hours since either of us had eaten anything, but I wasn't hungry. Finally, around 8:00 p.m. our family doctor arrived accompanied by a pre-med student. Together they examined Stacy. Jovial, our doctor agreed with the previous night's diagnosis and released Stacy with a boisterous high-five and a prescription for Vicodin. She told me to stop by her office the following morning for some samples of a migraine medication she wanted Stacy to try and information for the neurological consult. We stopped at the Wal-Mart pharmacy on the way home. Stacy waited in the car while I filled the Vicodin prescription. I was going through the motions because I was so apprehensive about the migraine diagnosis. Something in my gut that I couldn't ignore told me there was more to this—a lot more.

Chapter 4

Blind Curves

We gain strength, and courage, and confidence by each experience
in which we really stop to look fear in the face.
You must do the thing you think you cannot do.

~Eleanor Roosevelt~

When my girls were young we often went into remote areas of Wyoming with their dad. An avid hunter of big game, he searched for new locations where he could pursue antelope, elk, deer, moose, or mountain lion. Our trips took us through rugged terrain and on barely passable wilderness trails. Stacy loved the view and the sharp curves of the mountain roads. She would wiggle in her seat, eyes closed, giggling with glee. She called the particularly abrupt turns "squeeners" because they made her tummy feel funny. She would laugh—a comical mixture of scream and squeal—until everyone was hysterical. What a kick in the pants! Life has never been dull with Stacy around.

When we arrived home from the hospital that night, I helped Stacy into bed. The ordeal had left her exhausted—she just wanted to sleep. I tried but couldn't relax. Something kept me awake. I could not shake the feeling that a piece of this puzzle was missing. Actually I felt as though Stacy's segment of this intricate mystery had been tossed aside and not considered part of the solution. I should have been relieved with the diagnosis but I was very ill at ease. It just did not seem right. Questions kept popping into my head. I tossed and turned, finally getting out of bed around 5:00 a.m. for a shower and some coffee. I called my parents. They offered their prayers and told me to stay in touch.

I called my office and said I would be in later than usual. Stacy would have to stay home at least one more day so I called the campus bookstore and the Office of Student Life. I drove to our doctor's office to pick up the migraine medicine and her referral for the neurologist. I did not want to delay scheduling an appointment. When I arrived at her office, the receptionist gave me some samples of Zomig but the doctor was not in yet, so the referral would have to wait.

Stacy was resting at home so I went to my office for a staff meeting. I organized the files for projects I was currently working on. I spoke to a number of people about what happened. A pre-med student stopped by to say hello. John and I often talked about his plans to become a doctor one day. When I told him about the migraine diagnosis he asked, "Was it a TIA?" Realizing I had no idea what he was talking about, he explained that a TIA, or transient ischemic attack, is a mini-stroke with the same symptoms as a full blown stroke. Viewed as a warning, a TIA usually lasts less than 24 hours and typically leaves no residual damage. However, it generally indicates a real stroke is likely to occur.

I admitted to John how skeptical I was. He said, "Mona, this sounds like a TIA to me. You need to educate yourself about this in case it happens again." *Again! Oh, my God, please don't let this happen again!* I took his advice and did a brief internet search on migraine, stroke, and TIA. What I found convinced me that what happened to Stacy was not a migraine. The stroke and TIA symptoms listed were exactly what she had experienced: sudden severe headache, difficulty speaking, impaired movement, and one-sided weakness.

I didn't have time to dwell on what I had read. Stacy called to say she was awake but felt groggy. She wanted to take a shower so I left for lunch earlier than usual. When I arrived home she had already showered and was lying on the couch. Unusually weak, her head and neck ached. I gave her one dose of the Zomig and put her to bed. I called my office and said I thought I should stay home for the remainder of the day to see how she reacted to the medicine. I puttered around the house—doing dishes and laundry. Late in the afternoon I noticed a message on the answering machine from the hospital business office. They had a question about Stacy's insurance. I decided to contact them the next morning.

About 6:00 p.m. Stacy called out to me from her bedroom. She was in horrendous pain—clutching her right eye and rocking back and forth. To my horror the same scenario was repeating itself! I knew our doctor's office was closed so I called the hospital and asked the operator to page her. She returned my call within a few minutes. I told her what was happening. She instructed me to give Stacy one of the Vicodin and call her back. Stacy moaned and begged me to take the pain away. I gave her the pill but it took almost an hour for the pain to noticeably subside. I called the doctor back and gave her a report. She told me to call her back in an hour. When we spoke again around 8:30 p.m., Stacy was restless but in less pain. She had not attempted to get out of bed nor had I tried to move her. The doctor told me to call in the morning but not to hesitate calling sooner if Stacy's condition changed.

Around 10:00 p.m. the process began again. Intense pain in her right temple and eye made Stacy writhe in agony. She begged me to make it stop. I called the doctor again and she told me to administer both Vicodin and Zomig this time. Stacy cried out in pain while I was on the phone. Desperately wanting to ease her discomfort, I asked the doctor if there was more I could do. She was curt with me and said, "If you can't do this, Mona, take her back to the hospital." Not wanting to seem incompetent, I did as I was told. I have reprimanded myself a million times since that night for not taking Stacy back to the hospital right then.

As before, the medication took effect in about an hour and Stacy fell asleep. I called the doctor and gave her an update. She told me to try to get some sleep and to call her if anything changed. Sunday night had been my last full night's rest. We had just passed midnight on Wednesday night. I was exhausted but afraid to sleep for fear Stacy would have another episode. I made a pallet of blankets and pillows on the floor in Stacy's room. I would start to fall asleep and then jerk awake. It was going to be another long night.

Have you ever experienced something so profound that it etches a deep mark, almost like a scar, on your mind and soul? Later, when you recall that moment, it is so heartrending you painfully catch your breath because recalling the memory is like opening an old wound. I must have fallen into a deep sleep there on the floor in Stacy's room. I didn't hear her get out of bed and go to the bathroom. I didn't even know she had moved until I heard the toilet flush. Jumping up, I ran down the hall just as she stepped out of the bathroom. Bathed in a halo of white light, Stacy appeared angelic, ethereal. I hugged her tightly and told her she had scared me to death. She laughed a little, hugged me close, and said, "Don't worry so much, Mom. I'm going to be fine."

I followed her back to her bedroom and tucked her in the way I did when she was a child. Lying down on my pallet again, I remembered the childhood prayer the girls said every night before they went to bed:

> *Now I lay me down to sleep;*
> *I pray the Lord my soul to keep;*
> *If I should die before I wake;*
> *I pray the Lord my soul to take.*

Thinking of their little voices repeating the lines of that prayer, I drifted off to sleep.

When I awoke the next morning around 7:00, I immediately checked on Stacy. She appeared to be resting comfortably so I did not wake her. I made coffee, took a shower, and read the paper. Around 8:00 I called my office and said I would not be in. I needed to stay with Stacy and get an appointment with a neurologist. Today we needed to find some answers. Neither of us could continue this way.

I called our doctor's office and left a message. While I waited for the return call, I dialed the hospital business office. I was surprised that they could find no proof of medical insurance for Stacy. Confused, I called the student insurance office at the university and discovered Stacy indeed had no coverage. Somehow during enrollment for spring semester, she had forgotten to select it. *Crap! What are we going to do?* I decided to wait until I knew more about the neurologist before tackling the insurance issue. First things first.

I went into Stacy's room to wake her. I wanted to talk with her to see how she was feeling. She moved slightly to one side but didn't wake. I waited about half an hour more and returned. She was still on her side facing away from me so I tried to roll her onto her back. She blinked and groaned but didn't really respond. I was concerned but not overtly at that moment. I assumed that she was just sleeping off all the medication from the night before. I told myself to try again in a few minutes. I called the doctor's office again but had to leave another message. I was becoming anxious.

When I tried to wake Stacy again, I forcibly rolled her over. It was then I noticed the pronounced limpness of her left side and the droopiness of her face. I forced her talk to me. Her speech was slurred—I could barely understand what she was saying. She tried to hold her eyes open but they would fall closed. *Oh, my God! Damn it! This is not a migraine!*

Reliving the terror of Stacy's previous collapse, I called our doctor again. The receptionist said the doctor was with patients. I was desperate to speak with her but she couldn't come to the phone. I needed to know what she wanted me to do. If I couldn't speak directly to our doctor about this, then I needed to talk to the neurologist. Something was wrong with Stacy and we couldn't wait. The receptionist finally gave me the information and said, "I don't know what you're so worried about. We faxed everything already."

If I could have crawled through the phone line and strangled her with it, I would have done exactly that. All I could say was, "Why didn't you just tell me that sooner?" Relieved that I had the neurologist's name and telephone number, I quickly dialed the phone. It was nearing noon by now and I worried that the office would be closed for lunch. Reassured when an actual person picked up the phone, I explained what had happened. The clinic was in Cheyenne—about an hour from us. When the receptionist asked if we could be there at three, I begged for something sooner but she didn't have any openings. I emphatically said, "We'll be there!"

I called Camy and asked if she could help me get Stacy into my car. I knew I couldn't do it by myself. I kept trying to rouse her but had limited response. Camy and her friend Ann Johnson arrived around 1:00 p.m. Together we managed to get Stacy out of her bed. She resisted so I tried to explain what we were doing. She drooled and could not fully open her eyes. Her entire left side was lifeless. Ann looked at me with distress written all over her face. Uneasily she whispered, "Mona, she's had a stroke. I'm sure of it!" I nodded but couldn't answer. I knew she was right but I could not make myself say the words this time.

I pulled my car onto the lawn by the front door and tilted the passenger seat back slightly. I threw some things in an overnight bag—a change of clothes for Stacy and me, a sweatshirt, my cell phone charger, my address book, and my Bible. I called Tracy at my office. She offered to go with me, but I refused. I could do it alone, I told her. She tried to insist that someone needed to go with me, but again I refused. Camy offered to come with me too, but ultimately decided she needed to stay in Laramie with Jordyn. She and Ann made a chair with their hands and carried Stacy to the car. When we left Laramie I had no idea how long it would be before we returned home. All I could think about was getting Stacy to someone who could help her.

The drive to Cheyenne seemed endless. I thanked God the weather was good. You never know what to expect during a Wyoming spring. Stacy's head lolled forward even though she was semi-reclined in the seat so I kept my right hand on her chest for support. I silently prayed, *"Please! Please! Just let us get there! Oh God, please!"*

After several wrong turns and a frantic call for better directions, I found the clinic. I parked my car on the curb at the front of the building and rushed through the sliding doors. An attendant with a wheelchair was right inside. I grabbed his arm, dragged him outside, and told him I needed help to get Stacy out of the car. We were barely able to get her into the wheelchair without dropping her. As he pushed her into the clinic, I parked my car into the closest open spot and ran to catch up.

Stacy was slumped forward in the wheelchair when I reached her. I stood behind it and held her up. We waited only a few minutes before a nurse called us in. Her name was Beth and she was very sweet. Stacy stirred in the chair and then vomited all over Beth and herself. Unruffled, Beth helped me clean up Stacy's face and lap. She said the doctor would be right in.

Dr. Reed Shafer strolled into the exam room and shook my hand. He was so calm and listened attentively to every detail. He had to physically lift Stacy's head to look at her—she couldn't hold it up by herself. As he began talking softly to her, she vomited on his shoes. I said, "This isn't a migraine is it?" He said, "Let's hope so."

Very composed yet stressing the urgency, Dr. Shafer said we needed to get Stacy to the hospital. Beth was instructed to call an ambulance which arrived within minutes. The paramedics loaded Stacy onto a gurney and strapped her body down. She was scared but I reassured her I would be right behind the ambulance. Dr. Shafer said he'd meet us at the medical center. I grabbed one paramedic's arm and said, "I will be following you. Do not lose me! I don't know where I'm going." He nodded.

At the hospital, I parked close to the ER entrance and watched the ambulance pull under the opening door. The spring sky was darkening and the evening air was cold. I hurried inside. The paramedics wheeled Stacy into an exam room. An employee motioned me to her admissions desk. I gave her all the pertinent information. When she came to the insurance question, I told her what I had learned that morning—Stacy had no medical insurance. She touched my hand and said quietly, "Don't sign anything." She walked into Stacy's room with her clipboard and asked "Do we have your permission to treat you, Stacy?" Stacy made a semi-verbal response. The woman said, "That's good enough for me."

We waited in the exam room until Dr. Shafer arrived. He immediately ordered an MRI. Since we had arrived in the middle of a shift change, there was only one technician available. I agreed to stay in the room with Stacy during the test in case she began vomiting again. If she did, we had to get her out of the MRI tube because she was too weak to turn her head to prevent herself from choking. I removed my jewelry and inserted earplugs. When the test was finished, Stacy was taken upstairs to the Intensive Care Unit. Dr. Shafer told me he would let me know when he had more news. I sat beside Stacy's bed and waited.

Chapter Five

Proceed With Caution

Hope is a thing with feathers that perches in the soul;
sings a tune without words and never stops at all.

~Emily Dickinson~

In the open area at the center of ICU, Dr. Shafer sat at the desk near Stacy's room. The nurses had hooked her up to several machines that were monitoring vital signs. Fluids and pain medication went in via IV. One nurse came to talk with me about advanced directives (otherwise known as living wills) and Do-Not-Resuscitate (DNR) orders. Stacy had neither. It made me feel ill to even discuss the subject. Resting now, Stacy appeared childlike. Hours passed. I called the girls and my parents. Everyone was worried sick. One of the nurses offered me one of the family meeting rooms so I could lie down. At first I refused, but as the wee hours of Friday morning came, I finally relented.

I dozed on a small uncomfortable sofa but jerked awake every few minutes. I realized the purpose of the room. It was the private place where families gathered while waiting for or just receiving news about their ICU patient. I wondered what the walls would say if they could talk.

My muscles ached from fatigue but I could not sleep. I went back to Stacy's room. As morning dawned, I had a visit from a member of the hospital's accounting staff. The bill for Stacy's care had already exceeded $5,000 and it wasn't even 8:00 in the morning. When I explained our insurance situation, the employee mentioned several options, including applying for Medicaid. She said she would put some paperwork together and get back to me. Since it was Friday, she said I may have to wait through the weekend. I didn't know what I was going to do, but somehow that seemed like the least of my worries.

Dr. Shafer arrived and gave me the bad news. Although I instinctively knew and had tried to brace myself, it was like a mighty blow to hear the words. The MRI had revealed the truth—a blood vessel had burst in Stacy's brain—she had suffered a massive stroke. All of her vital signs were stable at that point but he was watching her closely for any changes. It was too soon to know what to expect. He said he would keep me posted.

I spent the day by Stacy's side. I called my parents, worried about how they would take the news. They were shaken but offered to help in anyway possible way. Mom asked if I needed them to come to Cheyenne but I hated to think of them traveling hundreds of miles across the state. I said maybe we should wait and see what happened. I really didn't have many details yet so I wasn't sure what to tell anyone. I called my office and gave Tracy an update to share with our department head and everyone else in the department. My co-workers were my work family and I knew they were worried too. Tracy emphasized that there was no need to think about my job—I had more important things to do.

My department head, Bernita Quoss, called me back. Sympathetic and supportive she said she would initiate the process for a Family Medical Leave Act (FMLA) request. I had accrued a significant sick leave and vacation balance over the years so I wasn't worried about having to take leave without pay. FMLA would protect me and my job during my time away from the university. We covered as many work-related bases as possible, talking about current projects and upcoming deadlines. She had recently made the decision to retire at the end of the academic year and I reminded her that it was right around the corner. We had worked together for several years—enjoying a mutually respectful relationship. The department would be under new leadership in the summer and I had been working diligently to ensure a smooth transition. Knowing I had the support of my supervisor lifted some of the weight off my shoulders. For now, I could take a step back and concentrate on the situation at hand.

Memories flooded my thoughts as I watched Stacy. She had been so full of life just a short time before. I knew in my heart that the stroke had happened sometime after our hug in the hallway while I slept on the floor beside her bed. I felt as if I had a block of ice in my chest. It was difficult to breathe. Seeing her so still terrified me.

I thought about all the silly things Stacy said and did. She was our family's little entertainer. Her imitation of Dana Carvey's character Garth from *Saturday Night Live* and *Wayne's World* was priceless. She could quote lines and entire conversations from movies and television shows. She always knew exactly what to say in any given situation to immediately lighten the mood and make everyone laugh.

Stacy loved the outdoors and was constantly searching for adventure of one kind or another. Recently she had acquired a passion for snowboarding. She bought a board and went to the nearby mountains with friends as often as she could. She had not mastered the sport yet but she was giving it her all. She had been that way since childhood.

Stacy and her sisters grew up playing outside in barns, corrals, and pastures. The wide open spaces were their playground. I never knew what they would find or what they would bring home. They gave me bugs, rodents, baby rabbits, kittens, puppies, birds, wildflowers and "nature" of a hundred different varieties. When they discovered something particularly intriguing, they'd march to the door together, and yell, "Mom, we found something we want to show you. Promise you won't scream!"

When the girls weren't in school, the four of them played together unless one of our neighbors' children came by with their parents. Camy took her role as the oldest very seriously. Wise beyond her years, she watched over her sisters and shielded them from family issues that were evident to her but not the younger girls.

Patty strove for perfection from early on. She hated the fact that no matter how old she became, Camy would always be older. She may have been second-in-command, but she mothered everyone and ordered them around like a drill sergeant.

Jeannie was the talker, the fixer, and the elaborate planner of whatever they were playing with. An avid bookworm, she read before kindergarten and simply willed herself to always do well. She gave herself no room for failure.

All three doted on Stacy. When she was a toddler, she never had to say a word. All she had to do was point at something and someone would get it for her. I used to joke about the fact that she never talked in full sentences until Jeannie went to school because she didn't have to.

Although all my children had accidents, Stacy was the one who took risks. When she was barely four years old, she broke her right arm. The girls had constructed a ramp by placing a board from the ground up onto one rail of a pole fence. They would run up and down—often jumping from the highest point. Not to be outdone by her older sisters, little Stacy followed their lead. This particular day she was wearing cowboy boots that were muddy from playing in rain puddles. She slipped off the board and landed on a rock. Camy dragged Stacy into the house, yelling for me. "Mom, Stacy fell and she says her arm hurts." When I tried to help Stacy take her jacket off, her tiny arm, fractured above the elbow, twisted grotesquely in the sleeve. She whimpered a bit but otherwise made no sound. The arm had to be surgically pinned. Stacy stayed in the hospital overnight. She wore a sling with her arm wrapped instead of casted so it could be checked periodically. It never slowed her down.

Stacy learned to pedal her bicycle long before she figured out how to use the brakes! Riding as fast as she could to keep up with her sisters, she simply slammed into the garage door to stop. Her daredevil ways didn't end there. She once tried to jump off the edge of a loading chute—easily 10 feet off the ground—using a plastic garbage bag as a parachute. She broke her left wrist when she fell off the hood of her dad's truck when she was nine. The list goes on.

Pretending to be a spy, Stacy crawled out onto the roof of the garage so she had a bird's-eye-view of the neighborhood. She nearly fell out of the huge cottonwood in the backyard more times than I can count. She was always the first one to shovel snow, rake leaves, hang Christmas lights, or jump on a ladder. In high school, Stacy was the manager of the girls' soccer team for three years. She competed in rodeo events—goat tying and cutting. She adored the little green Jeep she drove, especially when she could take the doors and hard top off and feel the wind in her hair. She was fearless.

I, on the other hand, was shaking in my shoes as I stood there holding onto my memories and gently rubbing Stacy's hand. I told her over and over again that I was right beside her. I needed her to know I wouldn't leave. I told her how sorry I was. I should have told everyone at the hospital in Laramie to go to hell and followed my gut feelings. I cried until I had no tears. How could I ever satisfactorily explain this to the girls? After they left home, it was just Stacy and me. It was my job to take care of her—to protect her from harm. I had failed the task miserably. I had let everyone down.

I was surrounded by my thoughts when I had a visit from Robin Chance, one of the hospital chaplains. Soft spoken and compassionate, she wanted to know everything about Stacy and the rest of my family. She took me downstairs to the cafeteria and bought me some lunch. I don't remember what we ate. She asked me if there was anything I needed. I told her I didn't even know. She asked if I had money. I had some cash with me and always carried my checkbook and debit card so I thought I'd be fine. She gave me $50 anyway—just in case.

Robin asked if I had a place to stay and I said I hadn't even thought about that yet. She told me about the lodging provided by the hospital and gave me a brochure. I promised I would check into it. She asked if I had clothes, etc. When I told her what I brought with me, she said she'd pick up a few things and bring them back. I protested, saying she really didn't need to, but she smiled and said, "Let me do this for you, Mona." She walked back to ICU with me, held my hands in hers, said a prayer, and left.

My mom called to say she did not want me to be alone. She had talked with my dad and several other members of the family, and they all agreed. She and my sister-in-law Gena were coming to Cheyenne to be with Stacy and me. She would not take no for an answer. I didn't argue. The truth was I was scared stiff and thought having some support might be good.

Later Robin returned with packages of underwear and socks, two colored t-shirts, a toothbrush, toothpaste, a comb, shampoo, contact solution and case, and a spiral notebook. Over lunch I had remarked about how I liked to write my thoughts down as a way of sorting through them. I had used that technique in my counseling sessions after my divorce and it had been very beneficial to my healing process. After she left I made my first journal entry:

> *It was a stroke. I was right but I wish I was wrong. I can't believe this is happening. Stacy isn't really conscious. She has mostly been out since last night when we got here. She sort of opens her eyes when I talk to her but doesn't really respond. She looks like she's sleeping—so small in the bed. Like a little girl. Lots of equipment. They are monitoring everything. They had to put in a catheter last night—she knew something was happening and fought a bit. Mom called. Gena is coming with her. They should be here tonight. I don't know much about what's going on yet or what we'll have to do. Lots of tests—MRI, new CT, blood. No real news yet. Will talk to the doctor when he comes back. I don't know what else to do. I am afraid to leave the room. It's my fault she's here. How can I tell her how sorry I am? This shouldn't be happening.*

I talked to the each of the girls several times. Camy planned to come over from Laramie with Jordyn the following morning since she didn't have to work. I asked her to pack some jeans and sweaters for me. Patty and Jeannie waited for me to give them more news. They would come home if I gave the word. Mom called from the road to say she had talked to my cousin and her husband who lived a few blocks from the hospital. They were on their way over to offer their help.

Two of the nicest people you would ever want to meet, Tim and Mary Kingston came into ICU with open arms. Mary and I had not seen each other in years but family can usually pick up where they left off. I knew it had to be unbearable for them to be there and put their own grief aside. Their daughter Hope had lost her brave battle with Hodgkin's about a year before. It had been a long fight with many months of hospitalization. She was just a few years older than Stacy. They offered their nearby home as a resting place. I agreed to spend the night, only if everything was still stable with Stacy, but really didn't want to impose. They told me I could stay as long as I needed to and gave me directions. I promised to call before I left the hospital.

Mom and Gena arrived about 10:00 p.m. I was so happy to see them. There's nothing like a hug from your mother when your world has turned upside down. My mother is the strongest Christian woman I have ever met. Together with my dad, their prayers have literally held our family together and guided each of their children through trying times. Most recently, Mom was caring for my youngest sister Lacey who had been battling breast cancer for more than a year.

Gena is married to my oldest brother Corvin. They are also a couple with strong Christian faith. Gena had been commuting for months between their home in Paisley, Oregon and Casper, Wyoming to care for her mother who was gravely ill. Gena is one of those natural caregivers with a big heart and open arms who steps in to help wherever she is needed.

I could not have asked for more supportive women than the two who came to my side. I was relying on their strength but could not confess my feelings of guilt. They both were tired after their long drive and insisted I also needed to rest. I would need to be strong for the days ahead, they told me. They offered to take me to Tim and Mary's. I finally gave in and agreed to leave with them. Nurses were attending to Stacy as they had been all day. I sensed no alarm so I told one nurse I was leaving for awhile. She had my cell phone number and Mary's home number. Maybe I could just close my eyes for a few minutes.

We quietly entered Tim and Mary's home and sat down on the edge of the bed to talk. The peaceful darkness was startled by the ringing of my cell phone. Thinking it was one of the girls, I was surprised to hear Dr. Shafer's voice. They needed me back at the hospital. Although the first signs of trouble were subtle, the situation had changed quickly and dramatically. Stacy's brain was swelling and she had lost consciousness. Her young life was slipping away.

Chapter Six

Teetering on the Edge

Yea though I walk through the valley of the shadow of death;
I will fear no evil; for thou art with me.

~Psalm 23: 4~

The brain is a miraculous organ. I added this information here because knowing how the brain operates when it is healthy can help you comprehend what occurs during and after a stroke. Encased inside the skull, resembling a withered gnarly walnut shell, the brain has three main parts: the cerebrum, the cerebellum, and the brainstem.

The cerebrum has two halves called hemispheres. The dividing line between them is called the midline. The right hemisphere controls the left side of the body and the left hemisphere controls the right. The two are joined together by a web of nerves—a delicate circuitry—that looks a lot like a map with crisscrossing roads and highways. Although each hemisphere has its own exclusive functions, together they compliment each other and work in unison. The cerebellum controls motor function, equilibrium, and posture. The brainstem holds the life source of automatic functions such as heart rate, body temperature, swallowing, blinking, digestion, blood pressure, and breathing.

Covering the surface of the brain is the cortex—a layer of vital tissue about the thickness of two dimes. This is what is better known as "gray matter." Think of it as the rind or bark of the brain—a protective coating for the inner parts.

The two hemispheres of the brain are divided into lobes: frontal, parietal, occipital, and temporal. Each lobe has a specific role. The occipital lobes process the images of the eyes and link them to memories. The ability to read and do math as well as enjoying the aroma and taste of your favorite foods are functions of the parietal lobes. Your appreciation of classical or rock music comes from the temporal lobes. This is also where memory is intimately linked to the sensations of touch, sound, sight, and taste. The frontal lobes control attention, abstract thought, problem solving, reasoning, judgment, initiative, impulsivity, inhibition, parts of speech, moods, emotions, and major fine-motor body movements.

The primary functional unit of the entire brain is a tiny cell called a neuron. The brain contains billions of neurons that act as little transmitters. Signals that pass through them result in every sensation, movement, thought, memory, and feeling. The brain is the most complex biological structure known to man. Stacy's brain with all of its separate yet conjoined parts was about to become the center of everyone's attention.

I berated myself for even considering leaving the hospital. I raced through the first door I saw. Later one of the hospital volunteers told me that the door I used was always locked from the inside after hours. It was a strictly enforced rule. No one believed that I had entered through that particular door. Located on the dark west side of the hospital, it was the only other entrance I was aware of other than the ER. I didn't take time to consider taking another route—I simply threw open the door and raced down the hallway to the elevator. I think a force much stronger than my maternal power opened that door knowing I needed to get inside. Someone was watching over me.

When we arrived back at the hospital, I called Camy. Apologizing for waking her, I asked her to drive to Cheyenne and call her sisters in Texas. They needed to hop on the first plane out of Houston. The situation was serious and they all needed to come together for Stacy.

Dr. Shafer was waiting for me. Mom and Gena were by my side. Tim and Mary came to lend moral support. Stacy's right pupil was dilated and there were other indicators of increased intracranial pressure. CT scans showed a midline shift. Dr. Shafer had summoned a neurosurgeon, Dr. George Guidry. Stacy was holding on by a thread.

Camy arrived from Laramie in record time with little Jordyn wrapped in a blanket. Dr. Shafer showed us the CT scans and MRI. The images are typically variegated shades of gray and white. When we saw the images of Stacy's brain, our eyes were immediately drawn to a huge black area in her right frontal lobe about the size of a potato or a woman's closed fist. I struggled to absorb what the doctors were saying. I have asked myself since if it is possible for the heart to freeze while beating inside your chest. If so, I experienced that phenomenon.

Dr. Guidry explained that in a healthy functioning brain, neurons never come in direct contact with blood. Blood flow to the brain comes through a maze of arteries and blood vessels. When a blood vessel bursts, as in Stacy's case, blood spews out into the surrounding tissue and upsets the intricate chemical balance of the neurons. As a result the neurons and their respective functions die. Toxic blood had been leaking in Stacy's brain for an undetermined length of time.

When the brain is injured, it reacts like any other part of the body—it swells. The difference is that the swelling brain is confined inside the skull and has no room to expand. The bottom line—the building pressure in Stacy's brain was compromising every part and every function. The midline was barely visible. The swollen tissue was pressing on her brainstem—her life source. Without surgery Stacy would die. Even with the surgery it was highly likely she would not survive. If she had any chance at all, the doctors would have to perform immediate surgery.

Dr. Guidry went on to explain the surgery in layman's terms. He would cut open Stacy's skull (craniotomy) to access her swelling brain and remove the damaged parts of the right frontal lobe and surrounding tissue (lobectomy). He would make a small hole about the size of a fifty-cent piece in the right temple area of her skull to accommodate the swelling.

Any medical word with "ectomy" means removal of something. Most of us know what an appendectomy or hysterectomy is—they are both fairly routine in these days of modern medicine. When I heard the word *lobectomy*, and realized that this doctor was telling me he intended to remove a piece of Stacy's brain, I felt sick. My stomach contracted. My heart beat wildly and felt as if it would leap out of my body.

I turned to the people who stood beside me for support. Mom and Gena, Camy and Jordyn, Tim and Mary joined me in the little room. I felt a twinge of that old adage "damned if you do and damned if you don't." I asked out loud, "How do I do this? She's dying! Twenty-one years is not enough. I want more time with her. I want to watch her grow up. She's not there yet. This can't be it. There's got to be more to her life!"

Mom held my hand and said, "When God gives you a child, He doesn't tell you how long you get to keep them." I knew she was speaking from the heart and from her dreadful experience of losing a baby daughter forty years before. The pain of her own wisdom was physically evident on her face. Tim and Mary were visibly dazed. Their eyes flooded with tears.

I asked Dr. Guidry about the piece of Stacy's brain he intended to remove. He asked, "What does Stacy do?" I said, "She's an artist." He shook his head and said, "She won't be able to do that anymore." As he continued to tell us about that area of Stacy's brain, we realized we were talking about more than the probable loss of body movement on her left side. There was also the likelihood of loss of sight, hearing, speech, and memory.

Based on what Dr. Guidry told us, we realized Stacy's right frontal lobe held so much of what made her the person she was. Her childhood memories, educational knowledge, and infectious sense of humor all lived in that part of her brain. That was also where her artistic talent resided. It was home to her ability to imagine what she wanted to capture on canvas, ideas for constructing a sculpture, and recollections of creative influences by her favorite artists. I could not imagine Stacy without those things. What kind of life could she possibly have? This man was telling me he had to remove that piece of her in order to save Stacy's life. He was going to take out what made Stacy, *Stacy*. How could I tell him to proceed? How could I tell him not to?

I asked Dr. Guidry what he would do if Stacy was his child. He said he actually had a daughter about the same age. I was shocked when he said "I would not do it. I would let her go." I couldn't speak. He said he saw this kind of thing everyday—people wrestling with decisions such as this. In his opinion, people needed to stop and consider the quality of life for their loved one. Part of me understood what he was saying but there was simply no way I could give up hope.

Having no personal experience with stroke or brain injury, I relied on my instincts as a mother. Dr. Guidry didn't know me or Stacy. He had no way of knowing what we had already endured. He knew nothing of Stacy's passion for life or our family bond. *What if he was wrong? What if there was a chance that the damage to Stacy's brain was not as severe as he thought? What if I said no and gave up too soon?* I owed her an attempt at saving her life. We would never know unless we tried.

Mom looked at me and said, "You have never given up anything without a fight." Fortified by her words I told Dr. Guidry, "We're going ahead with this. I think you're wrong. We're not giving up. Stacy can't fight for herself so we have to fight for her. There's so much she wants to do. We need to do everything we can to give her that chance. We'll take her. Whatever is there, whatever she has left. We'll take it and work with it. We need to try." Everyone agreed.

A chaplain arrived. His name was Glen and he came to pray for Stacy. I would have preferred to have Robin but she was not on call and we couldn't wait. We all went into Stacy's room together. Dr. Shafer gently told us to say whatever we needed to express. This was that moment you see depicted in movies—the final words to a loved one on their death bed. Trust me when I say nothing can measure up to the reality of knowing you could be speaking to your child for the last time.

Mom and Gena whispered another prayer together while they held hands and kissed Stacy's forehead. I asked everyone to leave the room except Camy and Jordyn. I dialed Patty and Jeannie's home number on my cell phone. They were waiting together for our call. I didn't wrestle with what to say. There were no secrets that needed to be revealed. The girls harbored no resentment of any kind toward one another. They simply didn't operate that way as sisters. They knew they loved each other and always had each other's back.

Camy and I held hands with Jordyn, the other girls listened in, and I talked to Stacy, speaking for all of us when I said: "Stacy, if you can hear us, we want you to know that we are going to fight for you. We don't think twenty-one years with you is enough time. We know you want to do so many things and we want you to do them. We don't care if you have an arm that doesn't work or a leg that doesn't work. We will help you and love you. You are the funniest person we know. You make us laugh. We can't imagine not having you with us. Honey, we want you to know that if it hurts too much and you can't hang on, we understand. We'll be sad if you can't stay with us but we'll be ok. We are so sorry this happened to you. If you need to go, we will let you. We love you so much kiddo. We'll be waiting right here."

Dr. Shafer opened the door and told us they had to take Stacy to surgery. One of the nurses was crying softly. It was an emotional ordeal for everyone. As they wheeled Stacy out of the room, I held onto Dr. Shafer's arm and said, "Take care of her. She's my little girl. This isn't easy for a mom." He patted my arm and said, "Mona, this isn't easy for a doctor." I felt hollow as she disappeared through the doors. It was approaching 3:00 a.m.

Numb, we settled into chairs in the waiting room. Someone found some pillows and blankets for us. Dr. Shafer warned us it would be a lengthy surgery. He said they would try to give us periodic updates.

I made a phone call to my former brother-in-law to ask for help in notifying the girls' dad. Under the circumstances, I hoped the sheriff where Neil was incarcerated would understand and grant permission for him to call us. The man had done few honorable things in his life but I was hopeful he would step up for his daughter's sake. He had been absent from our lives for several years. He was a stranger to us now but, as Stacy's father, I thought he had a right to know.

Jordyn crawled up on my lap. Wise for eight years old, she was trying to understand what was happening around her. Inquisitive, she had listened to the adult conversations. Her beautiful brown eyes huge with concern, she quietly asked me, "Grandma, is Stacy going to die?" I held her close and tried to reassure her, "Oh, honey, we hope not. The doctors are going to do everything they can for Stacy" Her little body and voice shook when she cried, "I don't want Stacy to die!" Her words broke my heart. I knew I needed to say something that she might understand. I hugged her to me as tightly as I could and said, "I know you don't, but honey, if God needs someone to paint heaven and He wants Stacy to paint beautiful pictures for Him, we would have to let her go there so she could do that." She nodded, wiped her tears, and rested her head on my shoulder. We cuddled together and waited for news from the OR.

Chapter Seven

Crossroads

Be strong and courageous. Do not be terrified;
do not be discouraged.

~Joshua 1:9~

According to Wikipedia, "it is challenging to define mother to suit a universally accepted definition, because of the complexity and differences of a mother's social, cultural, and religious definitions and roles." I don't believe mothers have any difficulty at all describing who they are and what they do. Being a mother has been the most awesome experience of my life. I would not trade motherhood for anything. In my opinion, being a mother is a combination of reward, renewal, and regret. Giving birth to a child can be the most remarkable event in a woman's life—thus the reward. Women worldwide know a personal meaning of a mother's love that is as unique as the individual. Watching your child grow and become their own person—a combination of mother and father—is renewal. Mothers sacrifice their health, wealth, and happiness for their children. They will go without food, clothing, and shelter to make sure their children have that sustenance. They will starve to ensure their child's survival—thus giving their own life and regretting that they somehow cannot give more.

While waiting for news about Stacy, I felt an intense need to do something. Unable to just sit and worry, I took a walk alone. I stood in what would be a new corridor of the hospital. Amidst the construction paraphernalia, I yelled at God and offered my life in exchange for Stacy's. "Please, don't do this! Take me instead. I will go willingly. You don't need her yet. Let her live life a bit longer. You can just take me." I begged to understand. *How could we be here? How could this be happening? How could someone go from being so alive and vibrant to the brink of death? Was I dreaming?* This was not real. It couldn't be.

As I stood there trying to make sense of the situation, I went back over each second since Stacy's initial collapse. I knew we had wasted precious time by waiting for our family doctor to respond. Brain cells were dying while we were waiting. Precious time lost—precious brain cells destroyed. We could get neither back.

Old habits die hard. Years of emotional conditioning in my abusive marriage had instilled in me a tendency to take responsibility for events that were in no way, shape, or form my fault. I turned the responsibility for what happened to Stacy deeply inward and blamed myself. No one else was there. It was my fault! I knew it was a stroke. I tried to tell the doctors in Laramie but they wouldn't listen. I should have forced them to listen somehow. I kept telling myself I should have tried harder. I had listened to the ER doctor who told me I was wrong. I tried to believe him but somehow I just couldn't accept what he was saying. As Stacy's mother, I should have shaken him like he shook me. I should have insisted more strongly. I should have done more.

In a frantic state I began asking myself what else I could or should have done. I could have insisted on more tests even though the ER doctor said no. *Would they have done the tests if I had continued to argue that it* was *a stroke? Could I have forced them to do a MRI? What about the second night when Stacy began experiencing the same symptoms again? I should have put her in my car and taken her to a hospital, but where? Should I have risked taking her back to our local hospital?*

Regardless of which way my questioning led me, I kept coming back to one place. I was to blame. My soul began to erode. My emotions imploded. I wanted to cry but tears would not come. I was afraid to allow anyone to see my misery for fear that they would know that I had failed. If Stacy died, I had no one to hold accountable but myself. If she died, I killed her.

I have never prayed such angry prayers. I wanted to take her place. No longer asking, I demanded that God take me instead of Stacy. I pounded my fists on the wall until my hands were numb. My mind was in a hysterical state—my thoughts riotous. *What if she dies? What will we do if she dies? Oh my God, what if she dies?*

I couldn't think straight. I can't explain why but I began wondering how to plan a funeral. I had never done that. I thought about what Stacy's death would do to her sisters. I couldn't bear the thought of their misery. Crumbling, I pleaded aloud, "Don't make us do this. We can't watch her die." Miserable, I fought the urge to run as far away from there as possible. I wanted to curl into a ball for some kind of comfort. In a last ditch effort to influence Stacy's fate, I angrily told God to either bring her through it or end it right there. I simply couldn't bear any more.

I forced myself to return to the waiting room. Jordyn and Camy slept. Mom was dozing. Gena was curled up with a blanket but got to her feet to hug me when I came back. There have been times when I have wished I could have been in the operating room to watch Stacy's surgery. I wondered what procedures the doctors actually followed, what measures they took, and what they talked about while they were inside Stacy's brain. It is nearly impossible to fathom what doctors actually do when they are working to save a life. Television shows and movies cannot possibly adequately portray the real thing. After almost five hours of waiting, Dr. Guidry appeared. It had been a grueling operation but Stacy had made it through. Our prayers had been answered.

We waited together until Stacy was moved from recovery back to ICU. Her head was tightly bandaged. She was on a ventilator and was hooked up to several machines that monitored different body functions. Although her face was slightly puffy, she appeared peaceful—like she was resting. The next 72 hours would be critical. Dangerous post-surgery brain swelling or bleeding typically occurs during that time. We wanted to avoid that. The doctors hoped she would gradually regain consciousness. As she did, they would be able to determine which functions were intact and which ones had been compromised. Although we knew time would tell, it was impossible to be patient.

Chapter Eight

No Guardrails

Faith is the substance of things hoped for,
the evidence of things not seen.

~Hebrews 11:1~

Nothing can adequately prepare a person for a tragedy involving potential loss of life. When crisis hits people react—often without thought or consideration for those around them. Their pain and sorrow are so great they sometimes strike out at anyone who happens to be nearby. No one can honestly say how they will act in response to a serious accident, illness, or dramatic event. We like to think we'll be strong, make all the right decisions, and say all the right things when the time comes but that simply isn't the case. We are only human.

The morning after Stacy's surgery we simply waited—too tired to do anything else. Mid-morning Camy received a call from their dad that didn't go well. Any hope we had that Neil would put his own feelings aside were dashed. Camy and I talked about how Stacy might feel and what she would want us to do. We were confident we were making the right choice by deciding not to call him again unless we absolutely had to. The last time Stacy had spoken to her dad had been when she was in high school He had been released from jail in Laramie where he had served six months on a drunken driving charge. He called our house and Stacy just happened to answer the phone. He asked her to pick him up and drive him to a friend's house several hours away. She refused. Admirably, she stood her ground and told him, "You got yourself in, Dad. Get yourself out." We had tried to do the right thing by informing him about Stacy's stroke and surgery. We trusted that Stacy would understand.

Patty and Jeannie were in route from Houston to Denver and then onto Cheyenne in a small commuter plane. They arrived about 12:30 in the afternoon. We'd had little contact during their trip other than a couple of calls to ask the question that a few hours before would have seemed ridiculous. "Is she still alive?"

Camy picked up her sisters at the airport and drove them to the hospital. I met them outside Stacy's room to warn them about what they would see. They had prepared for the worst so they were relieved to see Stacy sleeping. When they walked into the room, we were able to give them a tiny piece of good news. We knew Stacy could hear. She had responded to simple voice commands from Dr. Shafer and the nurses. We were so thankful that she could respond to sound. Patty wrote about her initial reaction.

> *The best way I can describe seeing Stacy for the first time is that the whole thing seemed strangely surreal. I just couldn't believe it. My little sister was so helpless, so fragile. There was nothing we could do to make the pain go away or to give her back the life she loved.*
>
> *Why? I kept asking myself. Why Stacy? Why would this happen to her? She is a brilliant artist who is on the verge of becoming a teacher. She has so much ahead of her. Why would it all come to a screeching halt now? She is so young with so much life left to live. Why?*

Dr. Shafer came back shortly after Patty and Jeannie arrived. He welcomed them and did his best to prepare us for the very real possibility of severe brain damage. Patty and Jeannie had talked to Stacy on Wednesday and had given her a hard time for scaring them with her initial trip to the Laramie ER. Everything had changed so quickly—it was almost impossible to believe. Dr. Shafer was able to gently rouse Stacy. It soon became evident that she could also see. We cried.

Dr. Shafer asked simple questions. "Stacy, do you know where you are?" She barely shook her head from side to side. No. Then Dr. Shafer explained, "Stacy, you are in the hospital. Do you understand that you're in the hospital?" She nodded ever so slightly. Pointing to me standing beside him, he asked, "Stacy, do you know who this is?" She made a slight movement. "Stacy, is this your mom?" Yes! Her nod was more pronounced this time. The fact that she recognized me was a promising indication that perhaps more cognitive functions were intact.

Jeannie moved closer to Stacy's bedside. The two of them were only eighteen months apart in age. Especially close, they enjoyed a unique kind of communication. When they were small they actually shared the same imaginary friends! Jeannie invented them but, while playing, she and Stacy both referred to these special invisible playmates. It was amazing! Jeannie wrote about her impression of sitting by Stacy's side.

I reached down, grabbed her hand, and said "Hey, kiddo." It was then that she opened her eyes and looked right at me. Our eyes locked and I think she knew something serious had happened. I could see it in her face that she was trying to make sense of why I had flown all the way from Houston. I felt so guilty; she was so young and had her whole life ahead of her. I would have given anything to trade places with her. I knew that she had to pull through this; her life wasn't finished yet. There were so many things that she still had to do. We had already gone through so much together as a family that it was not time for her to go. I never could have imagined life without her. In fact, life without her was not an option.

Jeannie sat on the edge of the bed while Dr. Shafer asked Stacy to grip his hands. Stacy could grasp with her right hand but there was no response from the left. We had been told to expect this. He performed simple touch and reflex tests. "Stacy, can you point for me?" She pointed with the index finger on her right hand. "How many fingers am I holding up?" She held up the appropriate number of fingers on her right hand. After only a couple of minutes, Stacy closed her eyes—exhausted by the questions and the examination. We would have to be patient a while longer before we would know the full extent of the damage.

Stacy drifted in and out of drug-induced sleep. It never occurred to us to discuss any "what she can't do" scenarios. We simply focused on what she could do. We had already decided we'd deal with the outcome—whatever it was. Each of us privately contemplated the situation but didn't share our concerns with each other at the time.

The nurses in ICU were fabulous. Stacy responded more willingly to one nurse named Kevin. She would actually smile around the breathing tube when he talked to her. We thanked him for his gentleness. The head nurse instructed us on the purpose of each machine. We learned to read body temperature, blood pressure, and heart rate. We watched the ventilator screen. The machine was set to take breaths for Stacy at equally spaced intervals. If she did not breathe, the machine did it for her. As the hours passed, Stacy took her own breaths more and more regularly—additional positive evidence that she was fighting back.

Everyone was emotionally exhausted, physically spent, and in desperate need of food and rest. Tim and Mary opened their home and we jokingly referred it as the Kingston Hotel. We agreed to regroup in the morning. One of the nurses found a small folding cot for me and brought it into Stacy's crowded room along with some blankets and a pillow. I stretched out on the cot—fully clothed. I couldn't leave Stacy in case she woke up, or worse, did not. No one argued with my decision. They simply let me stay. No further explanation was necessary.

The next day, Sunday, visitors from Laramie came to offer consolation. No one could make sense of this tragedy. The outpouring of support and encouragement was so touching. Dozens of cards were delivered. Everyone wanted to help but we had to ask them to wait until we knew what we needed. We monitored the length of visits and number of visitors. People brought fruit baskets, gift cards, flowers, and balloons. The words of love and support kept us from falling apart completely. We knew we weren't alone.

We were instructed to "stay close." It was way too early in the game to predict an outcome. Someone from our family was with Stacy every second. We never left her alone. We all agreed it was important that someone she recognized be there if she woke. Looking back, I realize we were given a lot of latitude in ICU because Stacy's condition was so unstable. Everyone involved in her care knew how quickly her condition could change.

Stacy would wake for several minutes and then sleep for hours. Her little body was exhausted. Her left side postured—a neurological term meaning she experienced muscle tension that pulled her head to one side and twisted her body. When I asked about that movement, thinking it was a sign of returning function on her left side, a nurse explained that it was involuntary and often an indication of severe brain damage. Hope shattered momentarily, I mulled over ways to explain this all to Stacy when the time came. She had no conscious awareness of what had transpired or that the left side of her body was paralyzed. I had no idea how I was going to break that news. How do you tell someone something like that? In Mom's journal, she wrote of that night. Her words spoke for all of us:

> *We sat by her bed and looked at this talented twenty-one year old girl with bandages all around her head, tubes all over her, and unable to move. Father in Heaven, be with Stacy tonight. We pray for her recovery.*

Chapter Nine

Which Way Do We Turn?

Anyone can give up.
It's the easiest thing in the world to do.
But to hold it together when everyone else would understand if you
fell apart,
that's true strength.

~Author Unknown~

In the powerful book, *Anatomy of Joy* by Dr. Jerome Groopman, the author—a practicing physician in the field of experimental medicine—wrote about valuable lessons on faith and healing that he learned from his patients. One lesson came in the form of a joke from a terminally ill woman that went something like this. It seems a group of saintly people were patiently waiting outside the pearly gates. Saint Peter checked each one's credentials very carefully before ushering them in. Suddenly a man rushed past, pushed the gates open, and entered Heaven. He was wearing a white coat and carrying a stethoscope. Someone asked Saint Peter why the man was able to enter Heaven before the crowd outside. Saint Peter replied, "Oh, don't mind him. That's just God. He thinks he's a doctor!"

During the initial 48 hours or so post-surgery, we met more medical professionals than we could keep track of. Some were kind and cordial while others were aloof and condescending. I think most people who have been in a hospital setting would agree when I say some members of the medical community don't have the best bedside manner. We tried to give them the benefit of doubt; after all, we weren't at our best either.

Stacy gradually became more alert although she was not totally aware of her surroundings. Weighted pads kept her head immobile. She was in horrible pain therefore medication was constant. She was justifiably confused. Since she couldn't talk with the ventilator in place, she tried to make hand gestures to tell us what she meant. She held Jeannie's hand and made a scratching motion in the palm. It took several minutes for us to realize she had an itch that needed to be scratched.

Stacy was visibly agitated and reasoning with her was difficult. When Dr. Shafer asked her to lift a finger and point, she was very selective about which finger she used! She felt the ventilator tube and tried to pull it out. She tried to remove the IV. We had to tie her right hand to the bedrail. She wiggled her hand around and around, bending her wrist at an odd angle until she slid her hand from the restraint. We had to tie it tighter.

By Monday afternoon, Stacy was stable enough to remove the breathing tube. She was very closely monitored. Pneumonia is always a concern when the patient is too weak to cough. She would suddenly have violent coughing spells that worried me but the nurses explained that they were necessary to the healing process. Without the ventilator breathing for her, she needed to clear any fluid from her lungs. I wondered how her little body could withstand the pain.

We discovered Stacy could move her mouth to form words although no sound came out. Inserting and removing a breathing tube can severely irritate the throat so we weren't overly worried at first. However, when a speech assessment was done it revealed the left side of Stacy's tongue, esophagus, and vocal cords had also been weakened—paralyzed by the stroke.

I had my first glimpse of her fighting spirit when Stacy spit out the numbing medicine before the speech assessment. The nurse was confused and tried to give her some more. She shook her head, clenched her jaws, and spit again. The nurse said, "I don't understand. It doesn't taste bad. It has a sweet banana flavor." Well, now her behavior made sense. She hates bananas! She wasn't just being uncooperative and obstinate. She was trying to tell us something.

Swallowing was nearly impossible for Stacy but also incredibly dangerous because of the lack of control. If allowed to drink, she could accidently inhale liquids into her lungs without even realizing it. She wasn't permitted to have anything by mouth. Dr. Shafer told us that with speech therapy she could potentially strengthen the weakened areas, relearn to swallow, and possibly regain her voice. Therapy would be started as soon as possible. We knew Stacy wanted to talk and that she was trying to communicate. We were happy with that for the moment—determined to help her learn to talk again when the time came.

I was summoned to the hospital's patient accounting office where I met Marilyn—the person who helped me initiate an application for Medicaid coverage. Upon meeting her, she informed me she was scheduled for official retirement in early May. She made it her personal goal to push everything through for Stacy before she left. The paperwork was staggering but I began filling out the stack of forms. The first step would be applying for Supplemental Security Income or SSI. Secondary was the request for Medicaid. Thankfully Wyoming's state Social Security office was in Cheyenne. We faxed the inquiry and awaited a response. Marilyn warned me that the final decision could take as much as 90 days. We didn't have the luxury of waiting that long. I prayed for a speedy decision.

Dr. Guidry came by to check on Stacy. I talked with him outside her room, remarking on her fighting spirit. He said, "I think you made the right choice." I was incredibly grateful that he had saved Stacy's life but it was all I could do not to kick him. If I had listened to him and not given my consent for the surgery, we would not have been having this conversation. He mentioned that we needed to discuss arrangements for rehabilitation when Stacy stabilized. He recommended a facility in Colorado—Craig Hospital—that specialized in treating people with traumatic brain and spinal cord injuries. I had heard of it and knew of a couple of people who had gone there. He said that it was one of the best rehabilitation hospitals in the country.

I felt compelled to tell Dr. Guidry about the lack of insurance and our application for Medicaid coverage. He quickly squelched the idea of Craig Hospital by saying "They won't take Stacy if she's on Medicaid. Craig is a private hospital." I asked if there was anything anyone could do—if it was the best place for Stacy then we needed to try to get her into that facility. What about other options? Who did we need to contact for more information? He must have noticed my obvious horror when he mentioned putting Stacy in a nursing home. He changed the subject quickly and indicated he and Dr. Shafer would make inquiries.

That day I sat on Stacy's bed and talked with her about what happened. She hadn't been able to ask questions yet, but I could sense that she was trying to understand. We had never kept anything from each other and I wasn't going to start now. Telling Stacy about her paralysis was the most heart-wrenching thing I have ever had to do. The memory of that conversation will be etched on my soul for the rest of my life. I could feel her heart breaking. She turned her head away. Her tears soaked the pillow. I assured her I would stay with her and always be there. We would get through this together. In my journal I wrote:

> *I can't find the right words to describe what happened today. I think a piece of my soul died. I told Stacy about her arm and her leg. Maybe it was too soon to tell her. She cried. Huge tears. She turned her head away from me and sobbed. I wanted to cry too but I couldn't. I told her we were going to do everything we could to help her get through this. We'll do it together. She'll never be alone.*

That afternoon we met Stacy's first physical and occupational therapists. I was surprised they would begin therapy so soon. They talked to us about how the brain can actually build new pathways after stroke. Initially they manipulated her body while she was in the bed. Her left arm and leg were totally limp. She could not move them at all. Two therapists moved her to the edge of the bed to sit up. She had no sense of balance. She would have toppled over had they not held her up.

Our support team of family members from far and wide came to help wherever they were needed. I sent them out shopping for a pair of high-topped athletic shoes for Stacy and strapped them to her feet to prevent foot drop. One of the therapists had warned us that foot drop occurs when paralyzed muscles can no longer lift and lower the foot. If the foot drops, recovery of that movement can be difficult—in some cases impossible. If Stacy had any hopes of walking again we wanted no obstacles.

Dr. Shafer and I discussed every aspect of Stacy's stroke. I was still very upset about the migraine diagnosis. He patted my hand and said, "Remember Mona, doctors aren't God." We all wanted to know what had caused the ruptured blood vessel that flooded her delicate brain tissue with caustic blood. He said she had an abnormal arterial tree in the right hemisphere of her brain that branched from the carotid artery. More testing would be needed to determine why the vessel was so small and what had caused it to burst.

I became obsessed with learning as much as I possibly could. What had caused the defect? What had caused the bleed? I remembered that student telling me to educate myself. I asked one of the nurses if there was a public computer available in the hospital. There wasn't, but she said she would ask if I could use one that occupied an empty desk in the ICU nurses' area. Permission was granted and I was allowed to use it when no one else needed it.

Whenever Stacy slept and I had a few minutes, I scoured the internet for everything I could find. My quest for knowledge and answers started here. For Stacy's sake, I needed to understand the terminology and learn to speak the language. I found an online medical encyclopedia. I wanted to know the meaning of every test, every term, and every symptom.

Computed tomography or CT scan uses x-rays to create cross-sectional layered images. Magnetic resonance imaging (MRI) can provide clearer, more detailed three-dimensional views of parts of the brain that are difficult to see clearly on CT scans. MRI can also show blood flow through veins and vessels. It can be used to determine the cause of headaches, vision problems, speech difficulty, muscle weakness, and to diagnose or rule out a stroke. Magnetic resonance angiogram (MRA) compliments the MRI by detecting malformations within even tiny blood vessels in the head and neck. *Wouldn't one of these tests have revealed the building pressure in the vessel if one had been done the night Stacy first collapsed at home?* I had requested a MRI. Knowing what that test could have revealed kept me asking why one had not been done. I kept digging.

What about the spinal tap or lumbar puncture as they called it? My research indicated the test is often used when a stroke is suspected, but should not be performed if there is any evidence of intracranial pressure because it can actually *cause* brain bleeding. *Did that test contribute to the burst? What about the medications our doctor had prescribed and I had administered? Why had Zomig been the medication of choice if the initial diagnosis was hemiplegic migraine.* The description of uses for Zomig indicated it is not recommended for that type of migraine. *Had it contributed to the burst?* The more I read, the more I wanted to know. I had more questions than answers and we needed answers. Stacy had a right to know what caused her stroke and I needed to know if it was my fault.

In one of my searches, I learned about tPA, the stroke wonder drug otherwise known as tissue plasminogen activator. Several people had asked me if Stacy had been given the "magic stroke shot." I had answered no, but wondered, if something like this existed, why it was not given to her. My web search found hundreds of positive testimonies for the use of tPA. The clot busting drug could, if used properly, reduce the damage from a heart attack or stroke. Nearly every reference to the drug's success cited the need for the patient to receive the drug within three hours. *Well, I thought. We certainly missed that window of opportunity. What if . . . ?* My heart sank.

I read about the different kinds of strokes. From everything Dr. Shafer told us, Stacy's stroke appeared to be the hemorrhagic variety. Only about ten percent of strokes fall into that category and there are several subtypes. I discovered that hemorrhagic strokes are more often fatal than other kinds of stroke. Also, more than half of the people who have a large hemorrhage like Stacy's die within a few days. *Oh, God! Now I know how truly critical these first hours are.* Every minute counted.

I read on. Survivors of hemorrhagic stroke usually recover some brain function over time, however, most do not recover all. *Ok, I thought, some but not all. Some could be what? Could Stacy rebuild enough of what she'd lost to live a semi-normal life?* We would not know that for awhile. Another item of interest was the fact that brain tissue heals ten times slower than any other part of the human body. Recovery, if we were lucky enough to begin, would be a long process. Now I had an idea of what we'd be up against if she made it through the next few days.

I asked Dr. Shafer new questions every time I saw him. When I asked, he explained that if a stroke is caused by bleeding (like Stacy's was) rather than clotting, drugs such as tPA can make the damage worse. I was so thankful for Dr. Shafer's thorough explanations. He too was searching for answers.

On Tuesday evening as I was searching the internet, one of the nurses came to me and said I had a phone call. I asked who was calling and she handed me a slip of paper with a woman's name on it. I assumed the caller was one of the girls' cousins so I immediately went to the nurses' station. When I picked up the phone, I was surprised to hear our family doctor's voice.

I really wasn't prepared to talk to her. I was still so rattled by everything that had happened to Stacy and had so many unanswered questions. I wrestled with the thoughts in my mind about whether the medical professionals in Laramie had missed or ignored the warning signs. She asked about Stacy. I told her that it *was* a stroke just like I thought. She admitted she was already aware because she had been contacted for Stacy's medical records. When she said, "I wonder if we should have taken her back to Ivinson [Laramie's hospital] that night," I nearly fell out of my chair.

I don't know how to adequately describe how I felt at that moment—angry, frustrated, humiliated, defeated, conflicted, and furious. It is more accurate if I admit I nearly lost my mind! I wanted to scream but my throat tightened. All I knew was I could not talk to her. Nothing she could say would fit with any element of what I was dealing with now. I resisted the urge to hurl the phone across the room and simply stated, "I cannot talk to you," and hung up.

On Wednesday afternoon, the sixth day in the hospital, Stacy was moved from ICU into a room on the Ortho-Neuro floor. Initially when the nurse told me Stacy was going to be released I panicked. I was so tired I wasn't thinking straight. I thought they were sending her home! Dr. Shafer was kind enough to explain that we were a long way from being ready for that. Stacy had stabilized enough to move into a less restrictive environment. He assured me it was a good thing.

Messages of faith and hope flooded in. Every time I read one to Stacy, I was touched by the choice of cards and the personal messages. One came from my brother Arlin who had fought a long battle with Crohn's disease. He knew what it felt like to have your life changed by something totally out of your hands. The card read, "Jesus is the Great Physician. He is watching over you—seeing to every detail. He loves you in tenderness, compassion, and gentleness. He will do His healing work. How good it is to know that you are under His special care. 'I am the Lord who heals you. Exodus 15:26'." Inside, he wrote,

> Stacy—Stay strong and remember that the Lord loves you and so do I.

My sister Lacey knew about personal tragedy from her year-long battle with breast cancer. The verse on her card was extraordinarily touching. It read, "Sometimes when we least expect it, life takes a sudden turn. Things are going smoothly and pretty much according to plan and, all at once, you have a situation to deal with. That is what you are doing now. I have no idea how I would feel or react in your shoes, but I do know this has to be very difficult for you. I want you to know that I'm here for you if you need me, pulling for you all the way and hoping for the best. Remember life also has a way of suddenly making things right. Just when you least expect it, a new door is opened, an answer is apparent, a situation is resolved." Inside she wrote a moving message of hope and understanding:

> *Dear Stacy—I thought this card said everything I was thinking. There were so many times when I was so sick that I was angry with God. I didn't understand why it was all happening to me. Why was He making my children see me that way? I know now that everything happens for a reason. Maybe He wanted me to be able to tell someone else (like you!) that everything will be ok. It won't be like it was before. It will just be different. I know I am stronger now than I was before I had cancer. I look at everything differently now. Stacy, just know that we all love you no matter what. Keep your chin up. I know you will be tough as an old boot, but remember it is ok to cry. You just cry all you want to. We all pray for you every day. God Bless.*

Chapter Ten

Steep Grade

When the world says, "Give up,"
Hope whispers, "Try it one more time"

~Author Unknown~

We were so glad to be out of ICU. Stacy's new room had a white board posted with all the pertinent information: her name, diagnosis, doctors' names, my name and cell phone number, and special instructions. The nursing supervisor met with me. Her name was Betty and she took an immediate personal interest in Stacy and the rest of us.

The room had a couch bed where we were a bit more comfortable while we spent time with Stacy. Mom and Gena felt safe to return home so they left on Wednesday afternoon. Stacy was settling in. One of the nurses found several soft knitted caps for patients who lost their hair during cancer treatment. She gave some colorful ones to Stacy. Her blond hair had been removed prior to surgery. The little caps would keep her bald head warm. Wednesday night I camped out in her room and was blessed with a relatively quiet night.

Stacy had a private bathroom with a shower so the next morning I quickly took advantage of the facilities and put on some clean clothes. It was Thursday. The girls arrived about 9:00 a.m. They were all so tired but ready for another day.

Stacy's therapists took her to the therapy gym. She was very weak but they helped her stand and guided her legs while she walked between parallel bars. They explained that it is often possible to trigger impulses and encourage the muscles to "fire" by forcing the weakened limb to move. Use of the affected leg is usually easier to regain than that of the affected arm. I noticed a full length mirror on the wall at the end of the parallel bars—directly in Stacy's line of sight. She briefly looked up and I wondered if the image registered in her mind. *Would she recognize herself?* She did not resemble the person she had been just a few short days ago. Her head was bandaged tightly. She had dark bruising under her eyes and her left arm was held securely in a sling. We had done nothing yet to prepare her for seeing herself this way. The short workout lasted only a few minutes. Exhausted, Stacy slept the rest of the day.

Thursday night marked my first full night away from the hospital since Stacy was admitted. I had been unwilling—emotionally and physically incapable—to leave her side. Everyone else recognized my fatigue but I would not give in to it. Taking pity on the rest of my family, Dr. Shafer kicked me out of the hospital and told me not to return until the following morning. Knowing my fear of leaving Stacy alone, Patty and Jeannie volunteered to spend the night in her room. Much as they hated to even think about leaving, they planned to return to their jobs in Houston on Saturday. I went to Tim and Mary's and slept for several hours. I don't think I moved at all once my head hit the pillow.

When I arrived about 6:00 on Friday morning, Stacy seemed different—restless and agitated. She was picking at the incision under the bandage on her head. A small trickle of blood ran down her forehead. I wiped it away. Patty and Jeannie had not slept well. They tried to sleep in shifts but they both had difficulty staying awake. They left to shower and nap at Tim and Mary's. Dr. Shafer came by on morning rounds. His examination of Stacy revealed nothing particularly unusual so he prepared to leave. He was actually leaving town that day for one of his clinic visits. When I asked him about how Stacy seemed different to me, he reminded me we would have good days and not-so-good days. This appeared to be one of the latter.

Stacy's therapists arrived and began working with her. We had some visitors from Laramie who lent moral support for her. Even with her own personal cheering section, Stacy was not responding well and was unable to do what she had done the day before. We concluded that there was too much distraction. The therapists agreed to come back in the afternoon to try again. The visitors were kind enough to leave.

I walked down to the lobby with one very special visitor. Leah Griffin had been Stacy's elementary art teacher and the person responsible for encouraging her to follow in her footsteps as an educator of young children. Mrs. Griffin was, by far, Stacy's all time favorite teacher. Stacy had done several college practicum experiences in Leah's classroom and volunteered there any chance she got. Leah was an especially dear friend. She was devastated by Stacy's diagnosis. We talked for about fifteen minutes then hugged goodbye in the lobby. I grabbed a cup of coffee from the kiosk and returned to Stacy's room. When I walked through the door I knew immediately that something was wrong.

I rushed to Stacy's side. Her pupils were fixed and dilated. She was sweating profusely. Beads of perspiration drenched her face. Her gown was damp. Her breathing was erratic and her face flushed. Her left side was posturing while her right side shook with jerky spasms. I couldn't get her to look at me. I buzzed the nurse and shouted that I needed help. I dashed to the door, found another nurse in the hallway, and literally dragged her into the room.

One nurse said she would call Dr. Shafer so I told her he had left town. A neurosurgeon, Dr. Steven Beer, just happened to be on our floor of the hospital with one of his post-surgery patients. He was strolling by Stacy's room when the nurse called out to him. He came in and did a brief examination. He mentioned that Dr. Guidry was out of town as well. He wasted no time in saying he was certain Stacy was suffering from a second hemorrhage and needed immediate surgery. She was crashing again. He rushed her to the OR.

I called everyone and told them to get back to the hospital. A nurse led me back to the waiting room that had been our family's haven just one week before. *Had it really been a week? Only a week?* We waited together—even more subdued this time. We couldn't comprehend that this had happened again. Everything had been looking up. We thought we were out of the danger zone. Stacy had been making progress and then WHAM! We felt very blessed that she had come through the first surgery. We had scarcely had time to wrap our minds around the fact that she had actually made it though that first night. She was so fragile. *How could she possibly survive another surgery?* The first one was touch and go. This time her brain was even more vulnerable. I knew the odds were not in her favor.

Dr. Beer came to the OR waiting room to meet with us. The surgery had taken more than five hours. It was late afternoon. He had performed a second craniotomy and removed more damaged tissue from Stacy's right frontal and temporal lobes. Jordyn sat on my lap as Dr. Beer explained what he had done. She reached out her little hand and held his arm. She asked him point blank, "Is my Aunt Stacy going to die?" Unflinching he patted her hand and answered, "I hope not, sweetheart. We're taking good care of her."

After leaving recovery, Stacy returned to ICU. One of the nurses was emotionally shaken by Stacy's story and told me how much it touched him personally. He had a daughter about Stacy's age. He shook his head and said he could not imagine being in our shoes. He was very patient with us. We worked with one of Dr. Shafer's colleagues in his absence. He advised us to stay close. I mentioned that Patty and Jeannie were scheduled to fly out the following day. He cautioned us with, "I wouldn't recommend it." We all knew what he meant—we were back to square one.

After surgery Stacy did not require a ventilator but she was on oxygen. She had been given two units of blood. One of the nurses remarked that Stacy's blood resembled red Kool-Aid when she first came in. She was hanging on by a thread. I spent the night in her room. I marveled at the remarkable treatment we received in those dark hours and was certain I knew the reason—Stacy was not expected to live.

Saturday we simply waited by Stacy's side. She roused more easily but kept her eyes open for only a few seconds at a time. She was in obvious pain so medication was constant. The following day was Easter Sunday. It seemed strange not to celebrate as we always had. There was no church service, no brightly dyed eggs, no Easter baskets, and no family dinner. It was a sad day for all of us. My mom and dad were at home in Sheridan praying for a positive outcome to this second round. Mom wrote in her journal about that day:

> We talked to Jeannie tonight. They are doing another CT scan because of pain. Stacy's left eye is still dilated. Oh, how we pray for this dear child. God in Heaven has promised to never leave us or forsake us. Dear Jesus, please stand by Stacy tonight!

Camy and Jordyn had to return to Laramie on that Sunday afternoon. Jordyn had been out of school for the entire previous week. Camy needed to get back to work after a week's absence. I hated to see them go but I understood. They were just a phone call away and we knew now, from experience, that they could be in Cheyenne in a matter of minutes.

On Monday I made a brief trip to Laramie in the afternoon while Stacy slept. Patty and Jeannie stayed with her. They would have to return to Houston the following day. They had jobs that needed their attention. While I was in Laramie I stopped at the university human resources department to finalize my FMLA request.

I stopped by our house. Everything seemed foreign. The Hot Seat sat in the living room right where we left it. I went into Stacy's bedroom, sat on the edge of her bed, and promptly burst into tears. I had been holding them in so they painfully gushed from my eyes. Crying left me feeling exposed and breakable. I allowed myself that momentary outlet and then pulled myself together. There was no room in this scenario for weakness. Stacy needed me and I had to be strong for her. She couldn't do this alone. I packed a few of her things including a sketchbook and some colored pencils. It was so bizarre standing there in her room knowing how much had changed since we were there last. There were reminders of her everywhere. Heavy hearted I returned to Cheyenne.

Stacy was restless and agitated when I returned. She couldn't fully understand what we were trying to tell her. Someone had sent a small basket of Easter chocolate. Knowing how much Stacy loved it, we asked one of the nurses for permission to give her a taste. Even now the thought of that small act of kindness stirs a touching memory for Stacy.

I wanted to have some chocolate. The nurse agreed to let me have a small piece. Patty broke off it and put it in my mouth. I had to suck on it. It had the most amazing taste—milk chocolate—sweet—melting in my mouth. It tasted so wonderful. I can't explain it still to this day.

Patty and Jeannie comforted Stacy in any way they could. They found a radio station that played her favorite country music. The bedside remote had an audio speaker so it was easy for Stacy to hear the songs. When Dr. Shafer came by he immediately noticed the twang of the singer's voice. Jokingly he asked what was playing. His next comment made everyone laugh. "If I was in the hospital and woke up to this, I would swear I'd died and gone to hell!" We weren't even aware of how badly we needed to experience another emotion other than fear.

On Tuesday, Patty and Jeannie returned to Houston. Everyone cried. Silent tears rolled down Stacy's face. The girls felt horrible for leaving. They had no other choice. Everyone was heartbroken. Stacy wasn't able to say anything to them to tell them how she felt. Not knowing what else to do, I lay down beside her and held her while she cried. Stacy and I were going to be alone now.

We had a visit from Stacy's friend Megan Shifflett. They had known each other since before kindergarten. Megan had made a soft red polar fleece blanket for Stacy because she wanted to give her something to remind her that she was thinking of her everyday.

That afternoon, as I sat by Stacy's bedside watching her sleep, I heard two women talking outside in the hall. We had noticed the other patients in ICU but knew virtually nothing about them. One young man had been injured in a motorcycle accident. We knew that much from conversations we'd overheard in the waiting room and hallways. He wasn't wearing a helmet and his injuries were severe. I recognized one of the women as someone who had been in his room. When she told her companion, "There are things worse than death," I did not completely comprehend her meaning. The young man never regained consciousness. He died in a room a few feet from us. I am not sure of the exact moment. I simply found his room empty a few hours after hearing the exchange. His family was gone from ICU. Over the next few months I would remember those words on several occasions.

By Thursday, Stacy was stable enough to leave ICU again and moved to the Oncology floor—a quieter environment with fewer patients. She and I became a team. Our family support was strong but it would have to come to us from a distance.

Chapter Eleven

Learning to Read Road Maps

*Be faithful in small things because it is in them
that your strength lies.*

~Mother Teresa~

Determined to expand my knowledge of how to properly care for Stacy, I learned as much as I could from the nurses. She was always cold and had a lot of pain in her neck and shoulders. One of the more helpful nurses showed me how to make little heat pads from small hand towels and warm them in a microwave in the break room. She also taught me how to help Stacy use the bed pan so we didn't have to call each time she needed it.

By the end of that second week, we had established a routine of sorts. I stayed with Stacy as long as I could every day but left her alone overnight while I slept for a few hours at Tim and Mary's. They made dinner for me and took turns staying with Stacy while I ate. I made myself a schedule: up at 5:00 a.m., shower, and arrive at the hospital around 6:00. I would grab a cup of coffee and a muffin or yogurt and fruit from the food court on my way upstairs. I stayed with Stacy throughout the day and did not leave until she fell asleep each night. Then I would go to Tim and Mary's for a few hours of sleep.

Stacy and I learned new words and their meanings: tone, ambulation, gait, atrophy, and spasticity. We discovered that paralysis does not mean total loss of feeling. Stacy's left side was hypersensitive. She couldn't bear to be touched. The delayed sensation felt like fire on her skin.

Hypertonicity or *tone* makes movement unsteady. Overly toned or tightened muscles are difficult to work with. Spasticity is the term used to describe what happens when muscles are continuously contracted. This contraction is caused by long periods of non-movement after a stroke and results in severe stiffness or tightness of the muscles. Limbs can be pulled into abnormal and often painful positions by spastic muscles. Stacy was in constant pain.

Muscle atrophy is a common problem after stroke. It is the loss of the mass of the muscle. In its worst form, atrophy is the complete wasting away of the muscle. Extreme weakness after a stroke results in the muscle tissue not being strong enough to hold the weight of the limb thus painful pulling on the joints occurs. Stacy was losing essential muscle on the left side. Her right side was overly tired from doing all the work. Her left ankle was too weak to support her weight and wobbled dangerously when she tried to walk. She was constantly at risk for turning it and causing significant injury. An ankle-foot-orthopedic device (AFO) was ordered.

The technician who measured and molded Stacy's left foot was an interesting man named Rick Jackson. The owner of a company that makes all types of orthopedic apparatus, Rick took a personal interest in Stacy. He talked with her about his own unexpected life-altering event in which he lost a leg in a freak accident when he was in his late teens. He told her about his long months of hospitalization and recovery. He was honest when he said how angry he had been and how he resisted all efforts to help him adapt to his changed life. He pulled up his pant leg and showed her his artificial leg. He joked with her about having different "legs" for summer, swimming, and other activities. Telling funny stories about his "one-leggedness," he made her laugh. He constructed her AFO himself with a Taz motif, her favorite cartoon character.

Another term we learned came when Stacy's left scapula, or shoulder blade, lost its ability to hold her arm in its normal position and her shoulder completely dislocated. Called subluxation, this is a common occurrence after stroke. The gap between her shoulder socket and the upper joint of the humerus was easily the width of two of my fingers. The subluxation gave her shoulder an eerie appearance. We had to constantly keep her arm in a sling to prevent further damage.

Our days were filled with therapy sessions, CT scans or other tests, and conversations with Dr. Shafer. Physical therapy included stretching and range of motion exercises that were an attempt to reduce the severity of the spasticity and atrophy. Adding insult to injury, Stacy started her period and developed a urinary tract infection. Dr. Shafer and I discussed the fact that the stroke could affect body functions such as her menstrual cycle. He said it was highly likely she would not have another one for some time. It was even possibly that early menopause would result from the trauma her body had endured. He reminded me that the majority of stroke survivors do not worry about their reproductive state. Most are well beyond their childbearing age. Stacy had remarked on numerous occasions that she wanted to have "a whole passel of little cowboys" someday. I decided not to break this news to her until we knew for sure it would actually be an issue. She had enough to deal with right now. We would cross that bridge when, and if, we needed to.

Stacy had frequent visits from her friends. She treasured them even though she couldn't talk and had to just listen to the conversations. She became an expert at hand gestures and facial expressions. One special visitor arrived with his heart on his sleeve and tears in his eyes—John Harrison, her high school soccer coach, presented her a with a team t-shirt. She loved it!

I received word from Marilyn that Social Security had scheduled a mandatory meeting with me to discuss Stacy's application for SSI and Medicaid. I was thrilled to know the process was still moving forward and had not stalled like others had warned me it might. Every day I chronicled our activities in my journal. My mom did the same. On April 24—Thursday—Mom wrote,

> We talked to Mona twice today. Stacy had a better day. She has been able to do some things that show she is improving. We are so thankful for answered prayers—God has sustained her through so much.

The next day her entry read, *Every hour of progress is a praise and answer to prayer.*

Gena came back to Cheyenne to help out wherever she was needed. Stacy did not want to eat—in fact she refused. Nothing tasted good to her. Her brain really hadn't healed enough for her sense of taste and smell to kick in. All food was pureed for easier swallowing. She detested everything on her plate. Gena was able to persuade her to eat yogurt, pudding, smoothies, and Jell-O. No one else could get through to her like Gena did.

Any liquid—water, juice, even Pepsi—had to be thickened so Stacy didn't inadvertently inhale it into her lungs. She drew the line at thickened milk. It looked like cottage cheese and she simply could not bring herself to try it. During one of her visits, Camy tried to encourage her baby sister to give it a try. She wrote about it like this:

> I remember giving Stacy a hard time about her not eating her food. She kept telling me it was gross and she just didn't like it. Being her big sister, I tried to show her it wasn't that bad. I took the biggest gulp of milk I could. It had a thickening agent added to it and let me tell you what it tasted like—uh, not milk!

Gena was so supportive and encouraging but more importantly, she made Stacy laugh. Together they spent hours watching movies on the TV in Stacy's room. I confessed to Gena that some of the nurses were more helpful than others. It seemed to me that Stacy responded better when the staff was upbeat and positive. Some were rude and talked around Stacy as if she could not understand them. They often raised their voices as if she was hard of hearing. They treated her like a child or simply ignored her altogether. Gena observed some of the same behavior and reinforced my decision to stay with Stacy as much as possible. She needed someone to make sure she was treated appropriately given her condition. It was great to know it wasn't just me.

Cards and letters came daily. With a family the size of mine, the majority were from my siblings, Stacy's aunts and uncles. My sister Loanna wrote,

> *Stacy—You are always in my prayers and thoughts. You're a great person with a lot of talent left. You have Cooper blood in you and we Cooper women are strong. Don't forget that we are all pulling for you and we're here for you if you need anything. Have faith that God is with you always and that together you can handle anything.*

My sister Callie took a humorous approach. One of her cards came with a list of things to do while in the hospital. Stacy's favorites were:

- Make a Halloween costume out of your bed sheets.
- Mix up a unique facial mask from your lunch. (This one was particularly funny to her considering her menu options and the strange pureed texture of her food!)
- Draw happy faces on your toes.
- Say the alphabet backwards. (At the time, Stacy couldn't remember the alphabet frontward so she laughed about this one!)
- Imagine what you'd say to customers if you ran an online dating service.
- See how long you can go without blinking.

Family and friends rallied around us even though they had to do it from a distance—we felt their support as if it were a physical presence. The mother and daughter journals that Mom and I were writing kept track of little milestones.

On day sixteen I wrote:
> *April 26—Stacy got to have a real shower today! We had a visit from cowboy evangelists Leroy and Reda Cowert. What a hoot! They made both of us laugh.*

Day Seventeen—Mom's entry:
> *April 27—We just praise the Lord today! Stacy got to go outdoors in the wheel chair. She is eating better and has some use of her left leg.*

On Day Eighteen—April 28, I wrote:

> *Gena had to leave. We hated to see her go. Stacy is really going to miss her. She cried. Gena and I cried too. During morning OT Stacy fell in the shower. Sarah [the OT] turned her back while Stacy sat in the shower chair and she slipped out. She couldn't get up and when Sarah tried to help her she got really mad at her and wouldn't let her help. Finally Sarah was able to get her up and back into the shower chair. She was wet and naked and kept slipping. She had bumped her head in the fall. I yelled at Sarah. She had told me to give her some time alone with Stacy so they could work on stuff. So I went downstairs to the sunroom for a cup of coffee. Sarah called my cell phone and I ran upstairs. If I had been there maybe it wouldn't have happened. Sarah was devastated. Maybe I shouldn't have been so harsh with her. But damn it, she needs to be more careful. Stacy could have been hurt.*

The afternoon after Stacy's fall in the shower, I had my first meeting with Social Security. It just happened to be scheduled at the same time as Stacy's transthoracic echocardiogram (TTE). The Social Security meeting was too important to miss because of what it meant to Stacy's request for Medicaid benefits. The test was significant too because it would reveal images of Stacy's beating heart and check for any abnormalities. Our friend Peggy Cooney came over from Laramie to sit with Stacy while I was gone and be there with her when the test was performed. It seemed funny to call her Professor Cooney so we rarely did. She had always been Peggy to us in spite of having served as Patty's faculty advisor while she was in college.

The meeting at the Social Security office was an eye-opener. While waiting to be called, I heard three different people pleading their cases to the receptionist. One needed help with filling out the "expletive" forms. The next never made it past his muttered repetitive comment of "it ain't right," but I was never able to determine what *it* was. The third, a man in a wheelchair, was so angry I momentarily thought I might need to hide. His benefits had been cut and he was livid. He ranted and threw pamphlets and other items all over the room. Such was my introduction to the agency I had come to seek assistance from.

Mike Allen was the man assigned to our case. Together we completed the initial request for SSI and Medicaid coverage for Stacy. I gave him Tim and Mary's address so we could process necessary documents more quickly. Camy came to Cheyenne only on weekends and brought my mail from home. I didn't want any delays in the process. Never condescending, Mr. Allen treated me with the utmost respect. He said he would be in touch and assured me the benefits we were requesting were there for people like Stacy who truly needed them.

Our search for answers to the cause of Stacy's stroke continued. Everyone wanted to know more about the abnormally small blood vessels in Stacy's brain. What had caused them to be so small? What had caused the burst? She had a cerebral angiogram on the nineteenth day. Angiography requires insertion of a small hollow tube into an artery; typically one in the groin area. The tube is carefully moved through the main blood vessels of the abdomen and chest into a major artery in the neck. The patient must lie still, not moving at all for the entire procedure and for several hours afterward. It was a long wait that took most of the day. Stacy was not allowed to eat until dinner that night and had to remain flat on her back the entire day. Her left shoulder and neck ached.

On the twentieth day, Stacy suffered from a horrible headache that would not subside. Nothing we did eased her pain. Her headaches had become more frequent and were increasing in length and intensity. Excess brain fluid had accumulated under the skin on the right side of her skull. It made her head appear grossly misshapen. Dr. Shafer and the neurosurgeons felt certain the fluid would re-absorb and the skin would adhere once more to her skull. To help make that happen, they tightly bound Stacy's head. It caused unbelievable pressure thus the headaches. She was miserable. The fluid contributed to her unbalance. She could not sit without leaning and toppling over. She had no sense of center. The chair in her room reclined so we were able to pad it with blankets and allow her sit there for short periods of time.

On May 1, we had another visit from Leah Griffin. She could always lift Stacy's spirits and brighten her day. They talked and laughed like girlfriends. Their bond was unique and special—Leah in her sixties and Stacy in her twenties. Leah desperately wanted Stacy to try to reconnect with her artistic side. She was certain it was still very much intact. She predicted Stacy's art would be an emotional and spiritual outlet during recovery. She suggested Stacy use a journal and sketchbook to record her progress.

Mom felt compelled to come back to help me out again, so my sister Loreen drove both my parents to Cheyenne on May 2. I was beyond tired and it felt wonderful to have Mom and Dad there by my side. When Dad entered Stacy's room, even the nurses cried. Cowboy hat in his hand, he bent over Stacy and kissed her forehead. His wrinkled calloused hand held hers and he asked her how she was. Old cowboys like my dad aren't necessarily known for their outpouring of emotions but Dad's feelings were visible for all to see. A man's integrity says it all for cowboys. Never claiming to be perfect, my dad has led his family through thick and thin. His faith in God has always been his guide. Everything he stood for came through loud and clear in that gentle exchange between grandfather and granddaughter. It was an incredibly touching moment. Collecting himself, he wiped his tears and hugged me. Knowing Dad, he and God had already discussed this visit and the outcome Dad hoped for. He and God know each other well.

Mom stayed for several days. She stood in for me so I could take care of some of the financial details of Stacy's care. She sat with Stacy for hours on end, reading to her, and trying to provide any comfort she could. The headaches from excess brain fluid were constant. One tactic the doctors tried was to use a needle and syringe to extract some of the fluid that had accumulated under the skin of Stacy's forehead. They held her as immobile as possible and literally sucked the fluid out. The process was incredibly painful. From an observer's perspective, it resembled an ancient torture ritual. Afterward, the nurses would bind Stacy's head tightly in hopes her skin would re-attach to her skull. She couldn't stand the tight wrappings. She pulled them off whenever she could, only to have them reapplied by the nurses.

Dr. Shafer brought us some positive news that we took with a mixture of hope and apprehension. If all the pieces fell into place, Stacy would be moved to Craig Hospital to begin rehabilitation by the middle of May. It was the best possible place for Stacy and they had agreed to take her. If she had any hope of leading an independent life, she needed the kind of rehabilitative care Craig could give her. It would be intense—much more structured than what the Cheyenne hospital could provide. Dr. Shafer assured us this was the best thing for Stacy.

Later, after Dr. Shafer left, Stacy started crying. She begged me to take her home. In a voice barely above a whisper—taking all the effort she could muster—she promised she wouldn't be a burden. "Please Mom. Take me home. Don't make me go there. Take me home. You can take care of me." My eyes stung with tears but I couldn't let her see me cry. I shook my head and said, "No. I can't, Stacy. I don't know how to take care of you yet. We need to learn how to do this together. I can't take you home. I can't." She cried and lay still—staring at the ceiling. Her image was reflected in the LCD picture screen up there that had alternating images of waterfalls, flower gardens, and other scenery. It was meant to add color to the room and give patients confined to bed something more appealing to look at other than the stark white walls. I wondered what she was thinking.

I made a trip to Laramie at Mom's insistence. I watched Jordyn play soccer and spent some time alone with her. She missed having her grandma and I missed her too. This was a big thing for a little girl to understand. I went home to rest for awhile. I had no idea when we would be able to return.

When Stacy had her stroke, she was only two weeks from finals, but we had missed the end of the semester and her exams. I had worked closely with the head of the Art Department to persuade two of her instructors to grade her for the semester based on what she had been able to accomplish prior to leaving. We had to process withdrawals from two other courses but the final instructor gave Stacy an incomplete or X grade. That meant she could finish the last few remaining course requirements when she was able to return to school and receive full credit for the course. Stacy accepted the alternative to losing all her credits for the semester.

The nurses allowed me to use a wheelchair to take Stacy outside and for other little tours around the hospital. One of our little walks took us to the hospital solarium. The solarium provided me with a resting place for a little solitude while Stacy was in physical therapy. Dr. Shafer insisted she needed to spend time alone with her therapists. It was critical that they build trust so she could feel safe when they were working together. I had an intense need to protect her. I had fallen, very easily, back into my mother's role and had reverted to the kind of extreme care you give a very young child. It was apparent I really needed to take a step back to allow Stacy to progress the way she needed to.

The solarium was quiet, warm, and comfortable. I usually curled up on one of the chairs and gazed out the windows. Spring was fighting with the remnants of winter but the countryside was gradually turning green. Trees were budding. Soon their leaves would add more color. The blue cloudless sky was breathtakingly beautiful. I felt so confined in the hospital—isolated from the outside world. I felt tethered to the building but knew I couldn't leave. I also knew I couldn't share that feeling with Stacy. I didn't want her to misinterpret my feelings as regret or annoyance. I could think of a hundred better places to be but none more important than where I was.

When I took Stacy to the solarium that day, I thought it might be good for her too. I chose the wrong day to do it. She was sad, angry, and frustrated. The pressure from the brain fluid made her nauseous and I knew the pain was awful. I had also noticed an increased level of depression. The visit lasted only a few minutes and ended badly. I poured out my feelings in my journal entry that night:

I took Stacy to the solarium today. I wanted her to feel the warmth of the sun and look out the windows. She didn't want to be there. She was very angry today. Therapy had been hard. I draped her red blanket around her, put one of the little knit caps on her bald head, and wheeled her upstairs in the wheelchair. The elevator scared her. When we entered the solarium she just sat in the chair and cried. We were the only two people there. I talked with her about going to Craig. I talked about having to withdraw from her ceramics class and art history. I told her I would do everything I could to keep her Jeep for her. I didn't tell her that there was probably no way she'd ever be able to drive it again. She sat and glared at me.

Finally she whispered the words she'd been holding inside. It was like a painfully quiet anguished shout. "Why did you do this to me? Why did you let them save me? Look at me? Why didn't you just let me die? I hate myself! No one is ever going to love me like this! I hate this!" She finally verbalized it. She hurts and I can't make it better. I told her I knew she was scared. I knew it was hard. But I also knew there was so much she would and could do. I hurt so much for her. I couldn't let her see me cry. I can't imagine how she feels. How can I help her? I think someday she will feel differently but what if that doesn't happen and she blames me forever? I hope she can forgive me. I did what I thought was right.

Chapter Twelve

Rocky Slopes

I am only one; but still I am one.
I cannot do everything, but still I can do something.
I will not refuse to do the something I can do.

~Helen Keller~

Stacy's intense headaches continued. She was wobbly from the pressure inside her brain. In physical therapy she walked in the hallways—a therapist on each side to guide her. She had grown particularly close to George, the sole male therapist. She worked hard for him and they formed a strong bond. When he left for a few days off, he sent a small bouquet of flowers to remind her to keep up the hard work in his absence.

Our friend Treva Blumenshine came by everyday on her lunch hour. She would make the most of her few minutes by doing whatever it took to make Stacy laugh. She also noticed Stacy's depression. It was hard to see her so down and not be able to do anything about it. Dr. Shafer prescribed an antidepressant but warned me it could take weeks to have an effect on her symptoms. She had every right to be angry and depressed after what she had been through.

Dr. Shafer and I continued our discussions on possible causes for Stacy's abnormally small blood vessels. She was tested for lupus, multiple sclerosis, and even moyamoya disease. Everything pointed toward a congenital abnormality. I asked about the difficult pregnancy I'd had with Stacy and whether that may have contributed. Early, before I even had a confirmed pregnancy, I experienced severe nausea and weakness. I bought and used a home pregnancy test but it was negative. My gynecologist prescribed some medication to initiate menses but it didn't work. He ordered more tests. Low and behold, I was pregnant.

The pregnancy was different from my previous ones and would ultimately be a turning point in my life. It reaffirmed my faith in God and my dedication to my children. A few weeks after the confirmation, I noticed swelling and bruising on my left foot. Shooting pain in my leg would wake me and keep me awake for hours. My obstetrician sent me to an orthopedic specialist who found a strange lump that he removed for biopsy. When the results came back, I was in my fifth month. Mom went with me to the doctor that day. When I heard the word *cancer*, I was shocked and terrified. When I asked about the baby, the specialist shook his head. He wasn't going to venture a guess as to what the recommendation would be. I left my children with my parents and traveled to Denver for treatment.

After meeting with cancer specialists at the University of Colorado Hospital, it was determined immediate surgery was critical. The tumor, a rare form of giant cell sarcoma, was growing at an alarming rate. The possibility of losing my leg was one thing. My life was at risk and along with it, my unborn child's life as well. The oncologists and orthopedic surgeons recommended that I terminate the pregnancy for my own health. One doctor even felt the need to remind me that I already had three healthy children at home. Trusting God knew what was in store for us, I refused to abort.

Together Stacy and I came through that surgery, although at the time I didn't know I was carrying another daughter. Severely weakened, but with my leg intact, I postponed chemotherapy until after she was born. When she was six weeks old, I handed little Stacy to Mom and went to Denver for the first round of eighteen months of treatment. Stacy's first year of life was spent shuffling back and forth between our home and my parent's. She came to recognize her grandmother as her primary caregiver and Mommy as the skinny one with the bald head.

I found myself questioning whether those life-saving procedures from twenty-something years before could have influenced what we were dealing with now. As we tried to find answers about Stacy's stroke, I remembered how ecstatic I was after her delivery to discover she was healthy. She had rarely been sick in twenty-one years. It was almost unheard of for her to take anything stronger than Tylenol. *Did my decision to see my pregnancy to term compromise my child's life as a young adult?*

Nothing the doctors discovered supported any firm conclusion. Everyone knew that something had caused the bleeding but what? My research told me that bursts such as Stacy's were usually caused when the blood vessel walls were weakened by heart disease or high blood pressure. Stacy had neither of those conditions. Prolonged drug use could also be a culprit. Again, that was not a factor in Stacy's case. *What had happened to weaken that blood vessel?*

I had to know if the steps that followed the initial diagnosis in Laramie had contributed in any way. I hired an expert to investigate.

Our last days in the Cheyenne hospital were spent in therapy and preparation for our move to Craig. Stacy was so frightened about going. A young physical therapist, not one of our regulars, mentioned that Stacy was "really in for it." She described Craig Hospital as boot camp and said Stacy was going to be in a totally different world. Her commentary really perturbed me and I wanted to shush her. Stacy needed reassurance not scare tactics. Those brief negative observations did more damage to Stacy's shaky resolve than all my encouragement could undo.

I met with Tracy Bennett, my co-worker and friend. She came to Cheyenne with every working file from my office that would likely need attention over the coming months. We prepared a calendar of anticipated projects and deadlines. It was a crash course in doing my job in my absence but she was willing to take on the task. She brought me a laptop computer for email and correspondence. Camy would come to Craig as often as possible so we planned to send work back and forth with her. It seemed like a good alternative and one that would keep me in touch with my work. Tracy sent a little card when she returned home. It read "God never meant for us to face the tough times alone. That's why He gave us each other." It was such a relief to know I had someone of Tracy's caliber to hand the reins to.

Speech therapy was Stacy's least favorite part of the day. The "hee-hee" and "ho-ho" exercises meant to strengthen her vocal cords made her feel foolish. I tried to lighten the mood by commenting that they reminded me of Lamaze training. The speech therapist said she suspected the state of aphonia, or loss of voice, was due in part to post traumatic stress. In one of our last sessions, she said something to Stacy about how the stroke must have been a terrible blow to her femininity and self-esteem. You should have seen the anguished look on Stacy's face! Until then we hadn't discussed her sexuality and what the future might hold in regard to dating or relationships. Well intentioned, I guess, the therapist suggested I give Stacy a makeover to boost her confidence.

After the session, I followed the therapist into the hallway. I thanked her for the suggestion but went on to say I thought it was inappropriate to suggest that makeup could fix this situation for Stacy. She had never worn makeup. It wasn't who she was. Stacy needed to know people could accept her as she was. That would be the only way to help her learn how to live with any lasting disabilities she might have. Pretending to make her something she wasn't would serve absolutely no purpose at all. The speech therapist stood before me—speechless. I asked her to refrain from making such comments in the future.

I was forced to stand my ground with other professionals too. Every time I encountered one of these situations, I was reminded of a conference I attended some years before. The participants completed an exercise to determine what animal they would be. After answering all the questions, I was the only one in the room who fell into the category of *female grizzly*. Laughing about it was easy because it was so true. I fit the profile like a round peg in a round hole. I knew I was the kind of mother who defended her "cubs" with deadly force but wasn't afraid to swat them when they needed it. Mama Bear was about to emerge from hibernation.

One nurse, unfamiliar with Stacy, waltzed in the room with the greeting of, "Well, what in the hell happened to you?" I pulled her aside and informed her that Stacy couldn't speak yet. I asked that she please treat Stacy with respect. The question was tactless. Stacy had been through an ordeal and was struggling to deal with it. "Read her chart," I told her. "It will tell you everything you need to know. If you want to talk to her, keep the conversation light." Later the nurse mistakenly tried to give Stacy solid medication instead of through the IV. Stacy couldn't swallow solids yet because of the choking risk. I blew a gasket! I demanded to see the nursing supervisor. It was unacceptable and dangerous—I would not tolerate it.

The next day I arrived to find Stacy sitting in the stench of an uncontrollable bowel movement. She was humiliated and kept apologizing. I asked if she told the nurse and she said, "She's mean to me, Mom." The nurse, yes, the same one, retorted, "Well . . . I asked her if she needed the bed pan and she said no." I ordered her from the room—refraining from pushing her the way I desperately wanted to. I cleaned up the mess, helped Stacy into a clean gown, and found fresh sheets in the drawer which I put on the bed. This time I insisted the nurse not be allowed back into Stacy's room. I may have needed to take a step back where therapy was concerned but no one was going treat Stacy that way.

We indulged Stacy as much as we could. She loved to be read to so every chance we had, Ann Margaret Manyak, her favorite professor, came to visit for the sole purpose of reading. She read *Holes* from cover to cover. Patty found and sent a copy of *My Side of the Mountain*, Stacy's favorite childhood book. I read to her nightly. She would lie still with her eyes closed and just listen.

Stacy began doodled in her sketchbook—strange little figures and shapes. I wanted to nudge her to do more but I knew she wasn't ready yet. Hopefully a time would come when she would want to. I bought her a journal and encouraged her to write in it. On May 8, she made her first entry. Scribbled down the right margin because she was unable to visually track to the left, words with letters missing, her first entry read:

> *Just laying here again lik always which sucks but I did go and walk som! So that's good . . . I guess. I leave for Craig on Tuesday but I am kind of scaried to go. I am afraid I will not make it. I know I*

*want to do it but I jus don't know if I can be strong any mor. Now
look at me no I am crying. What a baby! I saw myself in th mirror
a few days ago . . . and it scaried me! I looked like Frankinstin! I
lay in bed and look up at the ceiling and see myself in th picture. I
look like hell. Now I know what it really means when someone says
"you look like hell!" I am only a shell of who I really was . . . crying
again. I will be back in 5. Treva was here. I am so happy. It is always
good to have friends here. I jus wis I could get the "hell out of here"
Crying again. Sorry. It will take me forever.*

Writing her feelings down seemed to give Stacy an outlet for some of what
she couldn't bring herself to say. The next day we surprised her with a small
piece of real pizza. Later, she wrote in her journal again. Her scribbled words
went on for pages because she wrote only a few words on the far right margin
of each page.

*I am back. Just eating som pizza which is not too bad!! Unlike the
other stuff I have been eating. I am still worried about Craig. I know
it is the next step to going home. But I jus don't feel very strong right
now. I jus want to be home in my own bed in my own clothes driving
my Jeep.*

*Only handle so much she can drive me insane. Get this done. Don't
know what else to say right now. I guess it rained a lot today so I feel
bad for saying that but it is true. She drive me crazy. She is always
so sweet all the time. I can only take so much sweetness. Does that
make me a bad person? I hope not!*

*What now? I am just sitting in this bed. Treva was here which is so
cool. Jus seeing people brighten by days I hope the rest of my day
goes okay! I don't know what else to do for today. I guess I will just
lay back and try to get some sleep. I hate having to go to bed because
I am all alone. It seems forever. I wish this was all over!! I hope so
soon. I hate this. Seems like it takes so long for it to be morning. So I
hate night time! Why does this kind of stuff happen to me? God damn
it! Sorry for saying that but right now I don't like God so much. He
always does bad things to good people so I am not all happy with
Him right now. I know my mom is not going to like that but I don't
like him right now. So damn you God and damn this whole thing. I
want to be better right now! Please jus help me get through all of this
crap. I guess I shouldn't have said that stuff about God. Sorry God.
I will not do that again. Well I will try really hard not to say things*

like that any more. So now I will jus lay here in our hands. Now I am crying again. CRAP! I hate this. I hurt so much. I thought you didn't leave the young and the sick behind God so what happened? I feel alone. Crying again.

Two days later she wrote again.

Saturday May 10 Still laying here in hell. I could no sleep at all last night. Plus I got sick and threw up. So that mad it even better. I really hate nigh time now. It is so long and boring. Plus there is no one here for me to talk to. Like my mom or family and friends. What am I going to do? I am still scaried about Craig!! But I am not sure why. I can do this right? Right. I'm strong but am I strong enough? Oh man, this sucks! If I could go back in time I would change this from never happening if I could. But it does no sound like ther was any way for this to not have happened so no matter what I would have to go through this hell.

We celebrated Mother's Day on our last Sunday in Cheyenne. Camy and Jordyn came over. Cards came from the girls in Texas. Stacy slept better that day. She seemed more relaxed. For some reason, that day I worried about all the decisions I had ever made as a mother. That night my mom wrote about the significance of the day:

May 11—Mother's Day—I pray for the mothers in our family today and for all good mothers everywhere. As I have watched Mona taking care of Stacy day and night, I feel mothers deserve a special prayer.

On Monday, May 12, we met with Dr. Shafer. He talked with us about what to expect from the rehabilitation protocol at Craig. It would be tough for us to say goodbye to him. He had been our rock and anchor through 34 days of ups and downs. He was emotional too. He had literally saved Stacy's life by rushing her to the hospital that day we arrived in his office. He stood beside our family when we in the midst of the dark early hours. Now it was time to leave his care and all that was familiar and safe. We needed to hold on tight to the extraordinary gift we had been blessed with—a future with Stacy in it. The outcome could easily have gone the other way and we knew it. We had a lot of hard work ahead of us if we hoped to help Stacy appreciate her survival and learn to live her life to the fullest. We were on our way.

Chapter Thirteen

Uncharted Territory

You may have to fight a battle more than once to win it.

~Margaret Thatcher~

Following the ambulance from Cheyenne to Denver was nerve wracking. The day was chilly for early May. The wind blew out of the northwest making our vehicles rock back and forth. I worried that Stacy was getting nauseous inside. I could see her through the back windows of the ambulance—attendant beside her. The driver was not very familiar with the route we were taking and neither was I, so I was glad I had printed directions from the internet the night before in case we were separated in Denver traffic.

The drive to Craig Hospital in Englewood took over two hours. The ambulance pulled into the patient unloading zone but there was no place for me to park so I circled the hospital several times to find an empty spot. I stopped by the admissions office to complete all the paperwork. It took longer than I thought it would, so by the time I arrived upstairs Stacy was already in her room.

She was short with me. Anxious and worried, she asked where I had been and what took so long. This was new territory for us and I knew she was hesitant but we *needed* to be here. Stacy had survived her stroke against incredible odds. It had nearly taken her life but we couldn't stop there. Surviving wasn't enough. We had to fight back. We needed to move forward and rebuild every possible brain function.

Stacy's room at Craig was a stark comparison to the plush one she in the Cheyenne hospital. No frills—just a couple of chairs but no sofa or comfy furniture. There was no place for me to stay overnight in her new room. She noticed that right away. There was just a bed and small bedside table. A small TV on a swivel appendage fastened to the ceiling would provide some entertainment. The room could have housed two people but Stacy was alone. Windows overlooked the lawn surrounding the hospital and the street below.

Our first impressions of Craig Hospital were mixed. I don't know what I was expecting from the infamous facility, but the atmosphere seemed very casual to me. Patients were wearing their own clothing and many of the nurses were in jeans and t-shirts. My first thought simple. *Maybe Stacy will be more comfortable here.* I pointed out a few of the differences to her but she didn't want to talk about it. She didn't want to be there. Tears were rolling down her face. In her barely audible whisper, she begged me again to take her home. "Please Mom, take me home. I won't be any trouble. I promise. Please, Mom. Don't make me stay here." It broke my heart but I knew I couldn't give in to her plea.

I stayed long enough to get Stacy somewhat settled in her room. I needed to take care of my own housing arrangements before the family support office closed for the day. Otherwise I would have no place to stay. Stacy cried. I knew she felt abandoned at that moment but there was nothing else I could do.

There was mail waiting for us when we arrived. My dad had sent Stacy a message of support.

> *Hello there, Stacy—There's a whole lot of things I would like to say—maybe to make you smile or make you laugh. We are just so thankful you are showing so much improvement. We are praying that one of these days soon you will be able to just walk out of that place. You know—that is possible! Don't you give up. Just hang in there and give it all you've got. I know you can do it. I remember some of the funny things you used to say like the time you told me I looked good in pink. God bless and comfort you. Love, Grandpa*

While I was away from her room, Stacy met her new physical therapist. Red haired and vivacious, Jean Milholland waltzed into Stacy's room and made an immediate positive impression. When I returned, Jean taught us our first PT lesson—safely transferring Stacy from her bed to the wheelchair and back again. She also introduced us to a new approach to walking. We were proud of Stacy's walking ability but Jean did not want Stacy to walk until she had completed her assessments. She said it was essential that Stacy develop a normal gait rather than simply walking for the sake of walking. She planned to re-teach Stacy to move as naturally as possible while gaining strength and functionality.

It was obvious we were going to learn a lot here. Our first lesson was that Craig Hospital took a team approach to rehabilitation. Stacy would have occupational, physical, and speech therapists, and would work with each of them in individual sessions twice a day. She would meet with a recreational therapist 2-3 times per week. She was assigned a family services coordinator and a rehab physician. A neuro-psychologist would be added the following week. Regular meetings would be scheduled where all parties would report on Stacy's progress. Our rehab schedule was set to begin the following morning.

Our first week at Craig was exhausting for both of us. There were new words to learn and new approaches to discuss. We met all the members of our new rehab team. Benchmark assessments were completed so they could chart Stacy's improvements over time. In addition to Jean, the new PT, Stacy had a new OT, Lisa Strahn. She talked with us about what she would do to help Stacy become more self-reliant in terms of taking care of her own personal needs. Stacy was too weak and unstable while standing to even attempt dressing herself one-handed, so Lisa taught her how to get dressed in bed.

Every night when I returned to my apartment, I tried to do the one-handed tasks Stacy was learning. As was the case with Stacy, it was incredibly frustrating for me, but I thought I could help her more if I truly understood what she was supposed to do. I felt I could possibly help her work through some of the problems she was having if I could show her myself. I recognized that I was sometimes overcome by the impulse to just reach out and help her perform the task—or worse, do it for her like I had when she was a child—but I knew I couldn't do that. I finally made an agreement with myself that I would not allow her to face a future where she had to have help dressing, bathing, toileting, or eating. She was going to be independent if I had anything to do with it. She had to learn to care for herself.

Speech therapy had been one of Stacy's least favorite rehab exercises when she was in the Cheyenne hospital. Jennifer Quinn, her new speech therapist, had a big job in front of her. She and Stacy had a lot of work to do. As with all the professionals at Craig, she was up to the challenge. Jennifer established an almost immediate bond with Stacy and made significant progress on cognitive activities in a very short time. I was impressed by her ability to hold Stacy's attention for more than just a couple of minutes. That was not easy. The damage to her brain had left Stacy with an attention deficit that made it difficult—sometimes impossible—to stay focused for long periods of time. Medication for attention deficit was not an option. The part of Stacy's brain that could have been helped by ADD drugs was gone. She would have to learn how to deal with this complex—and annoying—problem. Jennifer Quinn was there to help her (and me) learn how to do that.

The other members of our team were Dr. Alan Weintraub and Kent Hamstra. Dr. Weintraub would monitor Stacy's rehabilitation and overall health. Kent would assist with Medicaid, housing, and all other aspects of Stacy's hospital stay. He would also be there to help me find necessary services for Stacy when she was ready to return home.

I talked to my parents every night. I gave them updates that they shared with everyone else in the family. Mom wrote in her journal about what we were learning:

> *May 16—Stacy dressed herself today. It took her 20 minutes. She wants to work on doing that faster. Mona transfers her from the bed to the wheelchair and then Stacy pushes herself with her right foot. Mona goes with her to the bathroom but Stacy is learning to do that alone too. She has been reading in speech therapy. She's really tired from all her therapies. Most of her mornings are spent in testing of one kind or other. She has lost 20 pounds. Her neck hurts—most likely from the brain fluid that isn't absorbing. She is progressing quite well.*

> *May 19—Stacy's throat is sore from acid reflux. She doesn't eat well and that is of concern to Mona. She has lost so much weight but she just can't bring herself to eat. Mona says the cafeteria food is wonderful. She hopes Stacy will eventually begin eating better. Stacy had her eyes checked. Her vision is good as long as she wears her glasses but she misses areas on her left. Mona has been able to help Stacy take a shower but she wants a bath! They will work on that.*

Cards and letters from friends and family helped us through the rough patches. Every day the mail brought positive reinforcement. My sister Loreen sent a card with a fabulous message that read, "You've been through so much lately and I know it has taken a lot out of you and at times it must seem like things will never be normal again. But I know that you'll handle it because you are one of the bravest people I've ever known. You might not see yourself that way but I do. You have an inner strength that keeps you hanging on in situations that would try the best of us. That's not to say that it's easy just that you're a fighter. Anytime in the days and weeks ahead that you need someone to remind you just how wonderful you are I'm here."

Inside she wrote:

> *I think about you every day and I mean that—every day. I wish I could be there, right beside you, helping you, encouraging you, hugging you. I would if I could. The whole family sends hugs and kisses (and that's a lot of hugs and kisses!!)*

Wyonda, my sister closest to me in age and my best friend growing up, struggled in search of the right words. Finally she just wrote what was in her heart as if she were sitting by Stacy's side.

I tried to come up with some great words and profound wisdom but you know that really isn't what I'm good at. I can say we all love you so very much and know that you have the inner strength and determination to come back stronger than ever. You have a wonderful network of family and friends and people you don't even know all across the country that pray for you every single day. I wish you could see the size of the crowd cheering for you. So every time you accomplish a new task, close your eyes and imagine us jumping up and down, hollering our silly heads off. That should put a smile on your face! I so admire your strength and courage. God brought you this far. He won't let you down now.

We wondered if we'd survive the new intense schedule. I missed Tim and Mary's companionship and reassurance. While Stacy was in her therapy sessions, I attended mandatory seizure training and learned what to do if that ever happened while I was alone with Stacy. I learned that seizure disorders are common in people who have suffered traumatic brain injury, including stroke survivors, and I needed to be prepared. Everyone talked with me about detaching myself so Stacy could learn to be independent. I already knew I had to do that, but I still felt singled out.

Tests abounded—CT, MRI, blood work, and Doppler. We met a new neurologist who talked with us about the excess brain fluid. He said another surgery might be needed to insert a shunt to drain the fluid. All I could think was, *"Not another one!"* We were exhausted but thrilled when Camy and Jordyn came to visit. We gave them a tour of the hospital and took some walks outside with Stacy in her wheelchair wrapped in blankets. She was constantly cold, partially because of the trauma to her body, but also because of weight loss and muscle atrophy. She tipped the scale at a slight one hundred pounds.

Treating people with traumatic brain injury (TBI) is one of Craig's specialties. The manual provided to all Craig patients and their families states, "Every 15 seconds someone in the United States sustains a traumatic brain injury. Every five minutes one of those people dies and another becomes permanently disabled." In our second week we met some of the other TBI patients and their families. That conversation I overheard in the Cheyenne ICU came back to me.

Two young women, both named Courtney, had been severely injured in car accidents involving drunk drivers. Both were in their twenties and had been attending college. Neither would ever experience anything resembling a normal life again. Dwight had been in a snowboarding accident. Although he was wearing a helmet, the impact of an unexpected fall on an icy slope nearly killed him and left him with memory loss among other things. Kaisa had fallen while rock climbing alone. Miraculously she was found by two hikers and airlifted to safety. Mike wrecked his motorcycle. He wasn't wearing a helmet. He did not recognize his mother or his fiancé. Brian had been in a car accident with several of his high school friends and hadn't spoken a word for several months.

Although each patient shared the common bond of TBI, no one shared stroke with Stacy. However, in the eyes of the parents, fiancés, and spouses I saw a reflection of my own pain and anguish. It was of some comfort to know I was not alone—someone else understood.

Our days were filled with therapy sessions and more discussions about the need for shunt surgery. The buildup of fluid interfered with Stacy's progress in therapy. She was constantly nauseous, dizzy, and off-balance. She was exhausted from the headaches. In spite of that, we reached a major milestone that week and shared it with the rest of our family. Stacy's voice had been gradually improving and finally, on Monday night, she talked to her sisters and my parents on the phone. Her voice was not strong. It was a bit gravelly but what a joy it was to hear her speak again. My mom wrote in her journal:

> We talked to Stacy tonight! She actually answered the phone when we called. What a blessing and answer to prayer.

One night after I left the hospital, Stacy fell in the bathroom and hit her head. When I arrived the next morning she told me about it and was angry at me because I didn't come right away when the nurse called me. The truth was no one had called me when she asked them to. I met with the nursing supervisor and asked to see the incident report. The rehab technician who had attended Stacy in the bathroom claimed Stacy fell forward and landed on her. If that had been the case, Stacy would not have hit her head. When Stacy gave the supervisor and me a visual demonstration of what happened, it was obvious the tech had been less than truthful. I filed an official request to have the tech barred from Stacy's room and insisted if Stacy ever asked someone to call me, they had to comply. I had hoped Mama Bear could rest for awhile but she couldn't quite yet.

A review team from Medicaid came to assess Stacy. I was at a loss because it was impossible to comprehend what it was going to take to actually obtain a disability designation. Sometimes we were treated with compassion and understanding, then they'd turn on us as though we had made it all up. It was inconceivable to think anyone would voluntarily do something like that! Bureaucracy is illogical. They observed Stacy in the therapy gym and spoke with all her therapists. Kent Hamstra took care of the majority of their needs. By the time they concluded their visit, we were assured of Stacy's eligibility—at least for eighteen months.

Shunt surgery was eminent and was scheduled for the coming weekend at Swedish Hospital adjacent to Craig. Our new neurosurgeon explained that he would insert the shunt into Stacy's brain and seal the open hole in her skull that had been made during previous surgeries to accommodate the swelling from the initial hemorrhages.

We met the hematologist who was studying Stacy's blood to find possible answers to our questions about the cause of her stroke. He explained that the blood is comprised of different factors. His analogy was that the factors are like ingredients in a cake—some more important than others. The first seven factors in the blood are the most crucial to overall body function. He had discovered that Stacy had a slight factor twelve deficiency, but concluded it was similar to having too few grains of salt in a recipe. It was not significant enough to have caused her stroke.

We had out first team meeting and discussed the upcoming surgery and predicted outcome. Plans were made for post-surgery therapies. Lisa would work with Stacy to learn more one-handed ways of performing daily activities. Jean would introduce the LiteGait, the standing machine, and the exercise bike. The two of them also planned joint sessions where they would work together to teach Stacy how to stand while completing simple tasks with one hand. Jennifer planned to use some computer games and writing activities to improve Stacy's visual tracking and memory. Stacy and I could barely conceal our excitement when Dr. Weintraub announced her projected release date of July 11.

On Saturday, Stacy had pre-surgery MRI and MRA. Loading doses of antibiotics and anti-seizure medications made her groggy. I walked along with her as she was transported through the tunnel between the two hospitals. We had come this way numerous times for the battery of tests she had needed since arriving. I waited while they prepped her and then spent the afternoon in a waiting room. By 8:00 p.m. the surgery was finished and Stacy was in recovery.

When she began to come out of anesthesia, she was in incredible pain. In surgery, they had used the same incision from her previous operations. This time however, they used staples to close it. Her head had been shaved again so her scalp was sore. Her head and neck ached. The shunt, a new model programmable via a small magnet behind Stacy's right ear, had been inserted and literally held in place with small screws. The drain tube ran beneath the skin behind her ear, under her collar bone, and down through her chest where it emptied into her stomach. When her brain produced too much fluid, it would drain via the shunt and be processed through her system with all other waste. She had a small stapled incision on her belly. A specially formulated paste of ground coral atop surgical titanium mesh formed manmade "bone" to fill the hole in Stacy's skull. Here she was recovering from the third brain surgery in 45 days. It was almost impossible to comprehend.

Pleased with the outcome of the surgery and not anticipating a need to keep her in Swedish Hospital, Stacy was released back to Craig. Therapy could not resume until Stacy recovered a bit more and she wasn't improving as quickly as everyone hoped. Her head pounded. The staples in her scalp felt like the edge of a spiral notebook. The incision itched and some of the staples were coming loose. She rubbed her head constantly. She had painful hiccups and vomited every time she tried to eat or drink. Urination was sporadic. We ran back and forth to Swedish for CT and x-rays of her head, stomach, and chest. Blood tests and Doppler ultrasound of her kidneys and bladder revealed an underlying problem—kidney failure in its early stages. The medications used to prevent seizure and infection during and after the surgery were too strong for her delicate system—it was shutting down. *Damn!* We made a swift trip back to Swedish—this time to ICU.

May 29 marked our fiftieth day in the hospital and what a day it was! We had come so far yet were once again face-to-face with a life-threatening situation. Dialysis was ordered and a central line inserted for ease of administering medication if the need arose. A team of renal specialists stood watch. Stacy's creatinine levels skyrocketed. Creatinine is chemical waste processed through the kidneys. Normal creatinine levels are about 0.6 to 1.2 milligrams. Stacy's were over 10! Her blood pressure soared. She drifted in and out. The narcotic painkiller Dilaudid eased her pain but gave her dreadfully scary nightmares. Stacy recalls that time with a mixture of humor and terror.

> *I had the strangest dreams. At one point I asked Mom about the big fat man I was leaning on. It felt like I was leaning into a large warm body that held me close. I had very weird dreams about Native Americans. I heard drums and everything. I thought the nurses moved me to a different place at night time—a kind of basement. I thought there was a fire in the hospital. I had a dream that Camy's face was melting off as she was popping up and down by my bed. It's funny that I remember all of that but not much of the technical stuff.*

In major cities, critical care units see a multitude of human tragedies. It was odd to be there witnessing the drama on one hand but also being isolated from it. One night a toddler was brought in. Details came not from the nurses and healthcare professionals taking care of him, but from the evening news. He had been viciously beaten by his father and didn't survive. I cried for him. Once more, Stacy and I were not far from death.

Stacy remained in ICU until her creatinine levels tapered off to an acceptable 1.3. After 10 days away, she returned to Craig on June 6, her twenty-second birthday. Everyone we knew sent a card, present, or flowers. The nurses and therapists welcomed her back and showered her with little gifts. The well wishers knew exactly what she needed—encouragement to keep moving ahead. The original exit date of July 11 was no longer realistic and had been pushed back indefinitely. We'd been side-tracked for awhile but now it was time to get down to business. We had therapy to do.

One card from my sister Myla had a simple statement on the front. "The distance is nothing; it is only the first step that is difficult." Inside she wrote:

> Dear Stacy—I know this birthday will probably not be your best but we know it will be special to all of us who have been so worried about you. I know it is hard sometimes, but look for God's purpose in all this because there is one and I know that when you least expect it, you will be the light in someone else's life. 'Rejoice in every good thing which the Lord has given you. Deuteronomy 26:11'.

My folks sent a special message in a card with these words: "You'll never know how often those who love you say 'I wonder how's she is and what she's doing today.' And you'll never know how often those who love you think of you and wish you their very best."

Mom's words—precious and heartfelt—gave Stacy a boost:

> I wish you could see the family "cheering section" wishing every day will bring some progress on this road to recovery for you. God bless you sweetheart. Happy Birthday!
>
> Love, Grandma Dorothy.
>
> From my dad, Stacy—I wish I could just wave my hand and make everything all right for you. But I will keep praying that real soon you'll be able to walk out of there. Never give up. God Bless. Love,
>
> Grandpa Jack.

Chapter Fourteen

The Long and Winding Road

Our greatest glory is not in never falling, but in rising up every time we fall.

~Ralph Waldo Emerson~

Hippocrates, famous physician and teacher of medicine, is said to have been one of the first to recognize the health benefits of physical therapy. The purpose of physical therapy is to identify and maximize movement potential while improving the quality of life. The therapists at Craig Hospital turned that purpose into practice.

It was such a relief to be back with the professionals Stacy had come to adore. She had missed them tremendously. She was incredibly weak and still very much 'under the influence' of the drug regimen she'd been on while in ICU. Weaning off the narcotics was not easy. Stacy had grown quite fond of the euphoria Dilaudid provided. She craved it and told Dr. Weintruab she'd "kick his ass" if he didn't give it to her. He told her about his work with inner city drug addicts who affectionately called the drug *dillydauds*. He knew how dangerous and addictive the drug could be. He refused to give her anymore and told her she was welcome to kick his ass whenever she could get out of bed to do it. She considered that a dare.

Stacy and I met together and separately with Dr. Jim Berry, the neuro-psychologist assigned to our team. It was his job to maneuver us through the emotional minefield of post-stroke recovery. He was also in charge of my "detachment therapy." In one of our sessions he asked me how I was holding up and I honestly answered, "Pretty well, all things considered." I don't think he believed me. He voiced his concerns about my ability to take care of everything

Stacy would need when we returned home and take care of myself as well. I told him, "I am ready to do whatever it takes. You need to know that this isn't our first rodeo. We've been in the dirt many times before this."

I was determined to help Stacy through recovery and rehab. While at Craig, we saw so many other patients with more serious conditions than hers. We recognized how fortunate we were. Our family dynamic of positive reinforcement and faith was holding us together while others around us were falling apart. One mother complained to me while we watched our daughters in their therapy sessions. The other girl was exactly Stacy's age. She had needed a tracheotomy after her accident that left a visible reddish-purple scar on her throat. Her head had been shaved like Stacy's. Our little girls had fuzzy new growth where their blond tresses had been. The mother told me her daughter had been concerned about her appearance. The woman's next remark shocked me. She said she informed her daughter that no, she did not look the same as she had before, and she never would again! I couldn't believe how brutal that comment was! My heart broke for the girl. She was already dealing with the aftermath of her injury and her mother was beating her self-esteem into the ground. I found it unpleasant and depressing to be around the woman so I avoided contact with her after that exchange.

A new patient arrived—a teenage girl who had suffered an aneurysm in the speech center of her brain. Her room was two doors down from Stacy's. When we noticed her with her mother in the therapy gym for the first time, Stacy remarked, "Oh, Mom. She's so young. We need to be their friends." Stacy's compassion touched my heart and it swelled with pride. What an amazing person! She was in a wheelchair, unable to move her left side, scarred, thin, pale, and fragile yet she exhibited empathy that far exceeded anything I had ever witnessed.

Each day we progressed inch by inch. We passed the days together and leaned on the support from our distant family. Stacy and I talked to my parents every night before she went to sleep. Sometimes my brother Arlin would be there to offer words of encouragement or his latest joke. Dad sang little songs that Stacy remembered from her childhood. Other times Mom and Dad sent little notes of encouragement. One from June 10 had a verse that read, "Remember as you recuperate that you're in the thoughts and prayers of others. 'They that wait upon the Lord shall renew their strength.' Isaiah 40:31."

Inside Mom and Dad wrote:

> Stacy—We just pray so much that you will be feeling better soon and that you'll be up and around. You have come through so many things. Every day brings new progress. We are so proud of you.

Almost everyday, I talked with one of my sisters. My brother Wade and his wife Janet sent their best wishes whenever they could. Corvin, my oldest brother, called daily. A long distance truck driver, he stopped wherever he was to make sure we knew he was thinking of us and praying for us. Everyone reached out to us. Patty and Jeannie sent cards or care packages. Camy visited every Sunday and took care of everything in Laramie for us. Mom and I recorded the days on our journal pages:

> June 8—I wrote: Stacy said she wanted to try to paint so Jean and Lisa took her to the rec therapy room. They set up a canvas and held her up while she tried to paint a tree. She was so disappointed. She didn't like what she painted but that's not important. This is huge! She painted today!!

> June 9—I wrote: Stacy's arm actually moved today! I was amazed! Thank God for this day and for the continued progress Stacy has made. Please energize her little arm and leg. Help her regain her strength.

> June 11—Mom wrote: We talked to Mona. Today went pretty well. Our prayers are almost like breathing now—we just feel like crying every time we think about Stacy. Bless her heart she's working so hard.

> June 15—I wrote: Stacy had a little card from Kevin [Patty's boyfriend]. He said he plans to propose on Patty's birthday. She said she's glad she's still here because she wants to go to the wedding. Smile!!!

We were delighted when a former Craig patient presented a special recreational therapy session. An artist before his spinal cord injury, he continued to create pottery that was some of the most exquisite I had ever seen. Stacy was fascinated by him. With his assistant's help, he used special adaptive hand tools to carve intricate designs in the clay. He talked with Stacy and encouraged her to keep trying. As he patiently showed her how he manipulated the clay with limited hand function, he told her she probably wouldn't be able to use a pottery wheel again with only one working hand but she could still work with clay in other ways. She listened intently to everything he said. He came back for a second one-on-one session with her. They made some small pots together. I was seeing brief glimpses of Stacy, the artist, fighting back. I smiled to myself. I wasn't going to draw attention to it yet. I would sit back and watch it emerge.

In mid-June, the girls' dad was released from jail. Neil had made no previous attempts to contact us so I was surprised when he called. The conversation did not go well. He couldn't grasp the reality of Stacy's condition and said, "Oh, she'll be fine in no time." He had no concept of what we had already dealt with or what we still needed to do. Stacy refused to speak to him.

Camy made a trip to Sheridan where their dad was living temporarily. His father, their grandfather, had left some items for each of the girls in his will so Camy went to collect them. She handled the situation as well as could be expected and told me about it afterward. She said she was tough on their dad and held nothing back when she told him to carefully think about what was best for Stacy. "Don't go, Dad, if you aren't going to be there for *Stacy*. If you go see her, you have to be sober and stay sober. If you can't do that, then stay away." He never came.

On June 21, Stacy and I waited patiently knowing Patty would be engaged by the end of the evening. Kevin planned to pop the question at dinner. Finally Patty called and couldn't believe we'd known all along. Stacy and I talked for a long time that night about the things she wanted to do: return home, finish school, drive, spend time with her family, and paint.

Stacy began to gain strength and was eating better. Whenever possible I would get permission from the nurses and take her for an outing to my little apartment or a local restaurant. We'd make pork chops, mashed potatoes, macaroni and cheese, or peanut butter sandwiches—comfort foods that she enjoyed. She would nap on my bed or we would curl up together and watch a movie. She improved enough to move from Craig East, where the more critical patients resided, to Craig West where patients were housed until they were discharged—the final step before going home.

Stacy's new room had a full size bed. What an improvement! She could stretch out and was learning how to roll over and sit up unassisted. Patty flew in from Houston for a visit. It had been almost three months since she'd seen Stacy so she was thrilled with the progress she was making. When she watched Stacy walking with a quad-cane, she cried. We spent the Fourth of July picnicking on the hospital lawn and watched fireworks from the roof of the building after dark. Patty was sad to leave but needed to get home to monitor the construction of the house she and Kevin were building. She hugged Stacy and said, "The next time I see you, you will be at home."

We met with our team again and were able to set a new departure date of July 25. Stacy counted down the days and pushed even harder in therapy. We went on group outings and thoroughly enjoyed an official Craig Hospital celebration called "Hobie Day" with the other patients. The annual event takes place at a local lake where patients and their families can ride in boats provided by local owner volunteers. Stacy drove a speedboat while I sat in the back. It was exhilarating! We had a little too much excitement. Shaken by the motion of the boat, Stacy vomited and had to return to the hospital earlier than everyone else. Regardless, it was a great day in the sun.

Stacy used the quad cane more and the wheelchair less. Her gait was improving thanks to the LiteGait, a training device that suspends the patient in a harness over a treadmill and reintroduces walking, while controlling posture and balance. Stacy really liked her sessions on the device. Jean, her PT, and other therapists surrounded Stacy and placed each of her feet exactly where they needed to be. Tirelessly they worked—session after session. To lighten the mood they sang silly songs to Stacy. She began referring to Jean as "Jean, Jean, the Dancing Queen." Her favorite 'Jean' song was *I'm a Woman* with that famous line, "I can bring home the bacon; fry it up in the pan . . ."

The two sides of Craig Hospital—Craig East and Craig West—are joined by a sky bridge over Clarkson Street. One of Stacy's early goals was to walk up on that bridge and watch the traffic below. We could see people on the streets and the little sandwich shop at the bottom of the hill where I went sometimes to buy cheeseburgers and root beer floats for the two of us. We both loved our strolls over the bridge and back again.

Stacy gained ground in caring for herself using one-handed techniques. Her left shoulder was still dislocated and painful. She had not strengthened it enough yet for the muscle to hold the weight of the bone. We were pleased with the small amount of movement she had in her elbow. She could lift her hand slightly from where it hung by her side. Involuntary movement was constant. She never knew how her arm would react. Loud noise would startle it. Once when she sneezed, she smacked herself in the nose with her left fist. We were determined to regain more movement and control.

One day when I worked on personal care skills in the bathroom with Stacy, we shared a moment that we still laugh about today. Having finished on the toilet, Stacy stood to pull up her clothes. She looked down to see that her left hand had a death grip in the elastic edge of her underwear and was pulling them upward into the worst wedgie of her life. It was a good thing she'd already used the toilet because we both nearly wet ourselves. We laughed hysterically until we had tears in our eyes.

Leah Griffin, Stacy's friend and mentor came to visit as often as she could and shared time with us in my little apartment. Stacy was particularly down on one of the days Leah stopped in. She was depressed and certain she'd never be the artist she had been. Leah gave her gentle but firm advice. "You're right, Stacy. You won't be the artist you were. Too much has changed. You will see the world through new eyes because you are not the same. Yes, you will paint differently, but Stacy, *you will paint*. I am sure of it."

July 18 marked one hundred days. I stayed with Stacy until about 10:00 p.m. As I was leaving the building for my apartment, I shared the elevator with a woman whose husband I had observed often in the therapy gym. His injuries from a mining explosion were severe. We made small talk. She mentioned that she had been watching Stacy's progress and remarked on how proud I must be. I told her about the significance of the day and how anxious we were to be going home the following week. She shook her head and said she hoped they'd be able to go home one day. It was number three hundred and forty-three for them. She'd left her life and family on the east coast to be by her husband's side while he struggled to regain brain and body function. They had been married for almost thirty years but their future was uncertain. I was humbled by her words and admired her fortitude. I knew how lucky we were that Stacy was making such amazing strides. I vowed to be forever grateful.

In one of her last sessions with Dr. Berry, Stacy talked about going home. She was afraid and anxious. So much had changed. She was worried about how others would see her. Whenever she cried in her sessions with Dr. Berry she would refer to it as "leaking." According to her, she leaked a lot. Previously he had gently offered the best advice he had to give, "Stacy, you may not have the full use of your body, but you still have so much to offer. You still have your sense of humor and you have the ability to love."

In this particular session, Stacy told Dr. Berry she had found some words to live by—Winston Churchill's famous statement, "If you're going through hell, keep going." Impressed with her ability to identify and relate to such powerful words, Dr. Berry encouraged her to go on. Never losing that infamous Stacy spunk, she told him she was also adopting a motto. She started to read it to him from a small piece of paper she had prepared, but couldn't keep a straight face and giggled out loud. She had chosen words from *Daily Affirmations with Stuart Smalley*, Al Franken's skits on *Saturday Night Live*. "Because I'm good enough, I'm smart enough, and, doggonit, people like me!" Dr. Berry could not contain himself. He laughed uncontrollably—totally abandoning his usual ultra-professional demeanor.

On July 25, after 107 days away from home, Stacy was released from Craig Hospital. She was so excited she couldn't sleep the night before. She was beaming when I arrived that morning. She said goodbye to all her therapists and favorite nurses. Dr. Weintraub and Dr. Berry came by her room and hugged her tightly. We headed home for the next leg of Stacy's journey.

Chapter Fifteen

Homeward Bound

Home is a name. As a word, it is a strong one;
stronger than magician ever spoke,
or spirit ever answered to.

~Charles Dickens~

Herman Melville wrote, "Life's a voyage that's homeward bound." Simon and Garfunkel sang about the same concept in their 1966 hit song. Nothing in lyric or prose could suitably describe our bittersweet return to Laramie. We left metro Denver behind and headed north toward the Wyoming border. When we left Cheyenne in May, the landscape was colorless. Now the beautiful green of high altitude summer was breathtaking. We'd been confined too long.

Stacy dozed a bit in the front passenger seat. My car was loaded with all my belongings, her wheelchair, and other miscellaneous items. When we pulled up to the curb in front of our house, we were surprised to see huge balloon bouquets. My co-workers had decorated the house, added a colorful "Welcome Home" sign, and stocked the kitchen. Stacy refused to use the wheelchair—she carefully walked from the car up the sidewalk to the front door using her quad-cane. I snapped a photo of the event. Stacy remembers it this way.

Walking up the sidewalk I cried like a baby. It was like I had never seen my house before. The smell of home still to this day chokes me up.

We were finally home. *Now what?* Before we left Craig, I called several offices in Laramie in search of a new primary care physician for Stacy. I could not bring myself to return to the one we had before her stroke. I found one who agreed to take Stacy on as a new patient and scheduled an appointment with him so the two of them could meet and become acquainted. We couldn't waste any time getting back into therapy either.

We decided to work with the outpatient rehabilitation clinic at our local hospital for physical and occupational therapy. They also provided limited speech services and weekly massage. We didn't want to lose anything Stacy had worked so hard to gain. Laramie didn't have a lot of options but we took advantage of everything we could find. I was apprehensive and I knew Stacy was too. She had bonded with her team at Craig and as a result she had gained strength and mobility. Without their dedication to her healing she would never have been able to return home.

This time Stacy's therapy consisted of sessions three times a week rather than every day. Her new team leaders were Kim Waters and Bridget Scholljegerdes. Stacy wasn't sure if she could bond again. These new therapists represented the third team she'd worked with and she was reluctant to "give" herself to someone new. She worried needlessly. They hit it off from the start. The setting for Stacy's therapy was much different that what she had become accustomed to at Craig. Her new "classmates" were easily three times her age!

Progress continued much the same as it had before. In one of the joint sessions with her OT and PT, electrical stimulation on her arm worked its magic. Her shoulder joint jumped back into the socket and stayed in place. In late August, Stacy sent the following email to Lisa Strahn, her OT at Craig Hospital:

> *Hello Lisa,*
>
> *it is me Stacy. I wanted to tell you the good news, I moved my arm today! I shook hands with my ot. my ot and pt did a co-treat today, I got on all fours and they did e-stim on my arm. so i thought you would like to know all about what is going on. next time I see you I will shake your hand!!*
>
> *I miss all of you guy so much, but I think I'm doing good!*

Lisa responded enthusiastically,

> *What good news! Thanks for sharing it with me—it is great to hear progress! Keep up the good work and keep me informed!*

I returned to work on a part-time basis and built a schedule that would allow me to work half days at the office and as many hours as possible from home. It meant Stacy had to be alone for a few hours each day. I used my work time at home to answer email and type correspondence or reports. I linked my office and home computers so I could access all my documents and files. Time in the office was used to assist students and faculty with whatever they needed. I managed to take care of everything I could and relied on Tracy to keep me on track when the juggling act became too chaotic. The readjustment was awkward for me. For months I had lived every second caring for and worrying about Stacy. I suddenly felt insecure.

We had lots of visitors. People stopped by with treats and offered to help with whatever we needed. My sister-in-law Gena came to stay with us for a few days. We had missed her special touch. It was our turn to comfort her—she had lost her mother while Stacy was in Craig Hospital. We could only pray for comfort, strength, and healing. It was impossible to take her pain and grief away.

My sisters Callie and Lacey brought Mom down from Sheridan for a long weekend. They were impressed with Stacy's progress. Mom was particularly glad to see how much function Stacy had gained during the months when she had been unable to visit. We also had a surprise visit from Jean Milholland, Stacy's PT from Craig. She had been camping in Yellowstone with her family and was on her way back to Colorado. She spent an afternoon with us and was excited about the work Stacy was doing with her new therapists.

Stacy's Aunt Holly from her dad's side of the family came to Laramie for a few days. We hadn't seen her in several years but were hopeful for an opportunity to rebuild a relationship with her. She was my girls' only contact with their Gupton relatives. Holly talked about Neil and said he was doing well after his release from jail. He knew Stacy was home but he never contacted us or made any effort to see her. After Holly left, she didn't either.

Friends in Laramie organized several different fundraising events and established a special bank account for donations. The financial assistance was beyond anything we could have imagined. We hosted a picnic to thank everyone who had supported us through our months away from home. So many people came that we could barely fit them all in our tiny house. It was a joyous occasion with so much to celebrate.

After four weeks home, Stacy decided to enroll in a one-credit-hour independent study course for the fall semester. She didn't want to put her education on hold. She feared if she sat out, even for one semester, she'd never go back. I adjusted my schedule to accommodate her therapies plus her class schedule. Still using a wheelchair for long distances, Stacy entered Donna Brown's classroom the first week of class. Professor Brown was one of her instructors from the previous spring semester who had agreed to grade her based on what she had been able to complete. She welcomed Stacy into her classroom as an assistant for her entry-level design course. Stacy never missed a beat.

In early September, we returned to Craig for a follow-up appointment. It was great to see the therapists Stacy had worked so diligently with just a few short weeks before. Our thoughts and hearts were still linked to these fabulous people. Lisa gave Stacy a less restrictive shoulder brace that supported the joint but allowed her arm to hang freely at her side. Jean worked with Stacy's leg and found it tighter than we had hoped it would be. It was becoming increasing difficult to put the AFO on. We consulted Dr. Weintraub. He suspected we might need a tendon lengthening procedure but did not want to rush it. We agreed to try other tactics first. Jean taught us some stretching exercises to do at home and gave us a list of more strenuous ones for her therapists in Laramie to use in their sessions. We visited with all of Stacy's former rehab team. We spent the day in the therapy gym but it was different for us now. Stacy was alumni—a graduate of the program. New patients had been added and previous ones discharged. The atmosphere had changed. Stacy hadn't written in her journal for a long time. She wrote in it that night:

> *I went back to Craig today. It was weird to go back to the place where I spent so much time. On the other hand it was really good to just be visiting and not having to stay there! Met with Dr. W. Saw Jean and she thought I was doing great! That's always nice to hear. I walked throughout the hospital . . . I don't know how far it was, but it seemed a long distance.*

Shortly after we returned from Craig, Jeannie called with frightening news. During her annual exam, the physician had discovered a lump in her breast. She was terrified. With my sister Lacey's breast cancer looming over us, we decided to take a proactive approach. It could be nothing or something malignant. We all needed to know. A needle biopsy was performed. Although the lump was thankfully benign, it was targeted for removal. There was no way I could leave Stacy and travel to Houston to be with Jeannie. Camy agreed to go in my place and serve as Jeannie's "surrogate mom." Jordyn stayed with Stacy and me. Jeannie came through with a small scar and renewed faith in family.

Wintery weather descended upon us in late September with an early fall snowstorm that closed roads and restricted travel. It vanished as quickly as it came, clearing the way for a beautiful autumn—my favorite time of year. Stacy and I had missed most of the summer so we soaked up as much sunshine as possible. In late October we added a family member—a tiny black and tan dachshund Stacy named Harley. The tiny dog wiggled his way into our hearts and onto the foot of my bed. Stacy had a companion to share her alone time at home. The two quickly became inseparable.

One warm afternoon we played with Harley in the back yard. Around and around the yard he'd race—long floppy ears extended like wings. He was adorable. Suddenly serious, Stacy turned to me with sadness and said, "Mom, I can't remember how to run. What if I can't ever run again?" She began to cry and went back inside. I didn't know how to respond.

We found a clinical psychologist to help us work through the transition of returning home and adjusting to the changes in our lives. Frances Price met with us twice a week to talk together and separately. She was amazing! We worked through Stacy's quest for independence and my role of allowing her to fumble through each step so she was adequately prepared to take care of herself. It was hard to let go but I knew how important it was for both of us.

Stacy was bonding well with her new therapists. Bridget took her to football games and to church. She refused to allow Stacy to think of herself as disabled. Yes, she had challenges but those could be overcome. In therapy Stacy was a favorite of the older clients who watched over her like mother hens. One elderly woman who'd also had a stroke talked with Stacy about someone she called Calamity. In her stories she blamed everything on Calamity. It took Stacy a couple of conversations with the woman to realize she was talking about her paralyzed arm not a person! Stacy laughed about that for hours. She decided to name her left arm *Esther*.

Increased tone in Stacy's leg and foot was causing pain and making it very difficult to do stretching and strengthening exercises. We had to use wide padded Velcro strips to hold her foot in the AFO. There was no way she could put it on alone. It was all we could do to relax her foot enough to squeeze it into the device together. A new AFO was made. Stronger straps were added to hold the stubborn foot in place. Her big toe was rigid and rubbed on her shoe. The toe became wickedly infected. We met with a specialist who removed the ingrown nail and cleaned up the infection. It was a painful procedure but Stacy was a trooper. We both understood that without something to decrease the tone, the same thing would probably happen again.

Stacy and I met with Dr. Shafer in Cheyenne for the first time since we left the hospital in May. He was so glad to see how much Stacy had improved. His nurse, Beth, greeted us warmly. Stacy sheepishly apologized for throwing up on her when she helped us that day. She hugged Stacy and said, "That's ok, sweetie. I'm surprised you remember that! I forgive you."

It was unsettling to be in Dr. Shafer's office again. I actually felt some anxiety when we pulled into the parking lot. Our last visit had been that day back in April when he met us for the first time. Memories flooded my mind. Dr. Shafer put us at ease. We discussed our frustrations with the lack of any real progress in speech therapy. The therapist assigned by the hospital was pushy and overbearing. Stacy felt undervalued. She did not respond well to the techniques used and was refusing to attend her sessions. Dr. Shafer recommended setting some boundaries with the therapist or finding someone else—reminding us of the crucial need to bond in a positive way with all professionals we worked with.

One warm Sunday afternoon, we made a trip to Lake Marie in the nearby Medicine Bow Mountains with Camy and Jordyn. It has always been one of our favorite places to go in the fall for family excursions. As expected—it was beautiful. Stacy wanted to hike on a steep downhill trail but didn't realize how difficult it would be. I had to let her try. We made it down together without much trouble but getting back up the hill took all the strength Camy and I could muster. We finally resorted to scooting Stacy up the mountainside on her behind because she could not walk at the angle of the slope. She ended up with dirt, leaves, and pine needles in her pants but we made it. She promised to more carefully observe her surroundings before she tried anything like that again.

After weeks of waiting, we received a summary from the expert I had hired to investigate Stacy's initial migraine diagnosis. In his professional, unbiased opinion, the doctors in Laramie had acted appropriately and reasonably in their care of Stacy. Although the treatment was not ideal—considering she was ultimately diagnosed with the stroke I had suspected—it was a fact that her symptoms had begun to resolve during her hospital stay. That supported their diagnosis not my gut feelings or mother's intuition. As hard as it was to do so, I had to let go of my anger. Bitterness would serve no purpose—it would only weigh us down. It would be counterproductive to Stacy's recovery. We had to keep moving forward.

Thanksgiving came on the coattails of bitter cold temperatures and a foot of new snow. It was beautiful! We rejoiced in all we had to be thankful for. We made plans to fly to Houston for Christmas. On December 4, Stacy wrote these words in the green brocade journal Jeannie had given her the year before. Her words—scribbled on the right margin, were getting closer to the center of the page.

It's been a long time. I had a stroke. Yes. I did but I need to learn that it will not get me down. But how? Where I'm at is just a stepping stone to a great temple of life. Not made of stone yet but of wood that can be taken down and made stronger later out of stone. I lie awake at night thinking if I will ever find love. I never found that rare thing before the darkness (the stroke). Will I be able to find it now? I've never had love in my life before. Will I ever be able to experience that? Or will I be lonely? It might not be so bad not to experience love in that form but it seems so sweet in the movies. But that's not real.

We spent the holidays in relative warmth in the new home Patty and her fiancé had built. Stacy did not feel well on the plane but soon found new inspiration at the Houston Museum of Modern Art. A special exhibit featured 200 paintings by some of the artists Stacy had studied but wondered if she'd ever see: Renoir, Matisse, Seurat, Mondrian, Picasso, Monet, Dali, and Pollock. She stood in front of Van Gogh's *Starry Night* for the longest time. She told us about each of her favorite pieces, the artists, the periods, and the medium used. It was amazing that she could recall such detail. She and I sat side by side on a bench and stared in awe at the *Water Lilies*—neither of us spoke. It was touching to see Stacy's genuine excitement and joy. The artist within her was rejuvenated.

The year ended on a positive note. We talked about all we had been through and how we were different people than we'd been just one short year before. The mere fact that we were all still alive was a blessing in itself but when we stopped to realize what that survival had entailed, we were certain we had experienced a miracle. We bid farewell to 2003—our most challenging year to date—and met 2004 with enthusiasm and excitement. We were moving forward at a slow but steady pace. My mom wrote in her journal about our remarkable year:

> *Another year has just slipped by and as we look back over it—God has been so good! The events that have brought us to our knees have made us more and more aware of our total dependence on our Heavenly Father. We are so thankful for answered prayers. Stacy is doing well—not perfectly recovered from her stroke, but when we remember how we thought we would lose her, we are so thankful and thrilled at the progress she has made. We just praise the Lord for every day we have together as a family.*

Chapter Sixteen

Mile Markers

If you hear a voice within you say "you cannot paint,"
then by all means paint,
and that voice will be silenced.

~Vincent Van Gogh~

The oldest known paintings in the world are in the Chauvet Cave in southern France. Images of prehistoric hunters following horses, bears, rhinos, and bison in varied shades of red, yellow, black, and brown roam across the ancient cave walls. Discovered in 1994 by three cave explorers, the paintings are said to be approximately 35,000 years old. They became one of Stacy's favorite examples of artistic expression when she first read about them in junior high. She often sketched animals in much the same way—abstract and primitive. I hoped she would begin expressing herself artistically and I didn't care what style she chose.

Gradually, reluctantly, Stacy ventured into her studio. She put a canvas on her easel. It sat there for weeks—untouched. One day when I came home from work, I noticed she had painted an awesome scene—rugged mountain peaks shrouded in fog—bold strokes in shades of blue and gray. I was thrilled and asked her when she planned to finish it. She seemed surprised that I would ask that question. She frowned at me and said, "It *is* finished." She left the painting on her easel. Every time I walked by I looked at it. The quality was exceptional. The colors blended perfectly to capture the subject. Everything about it was magnificent. The solitary flaw, if you could dare to call it that, was that it was painted on only half the canvas—the left half was almost completely blank. Stacy's brain did not register her left visual deficit. I wanted to see if she would recognize it on her own later so I kept silent.

In mid-January 2004 we returned to Craig for re-evaluation. We spent time in the Spasticity Clinic in hopes of finding some way to work with the increased tone in Stacy's left leg. She had long since abandoned the wheelchair and quad cane for a simple black cane that she decorated with silly stickers. Phenol injections were our first option but led to no relief. Several weeks later we tried Botox. Stacy joked about never having to worry about wrinkly knees! We had some relief with the Botox so tried again, but in the end Stacy's doctors decided tendon lengthening surgery would be our best bet.

We found a surgeon, Dr. Roger Sobel, at the Orthopedic Center of the Rockies in Fort Collins, Colorado. He and Stacy instantly formed a bond. In March he performed the delicate Z-cut surgery on Stacy's Achilles tendon and a similar loosening of the tight ones in her big toe. Encased in a colorful pink tie-dyed cast, her leg healed well and the muscles relaxed. She said goodbye to her AFO and began using a simple ankle wrap.

On April 10, surrounded by family and friends, Stacy celebrated one year of stroke survival. Our house was filled to capacity. We toasted her success and determination. One of our guests was Leah Griffin, Stacy's friend and mentor. I took her into Stacy's studio and showed her the painting of the mountains. She was awestruck as I had been. I told her, "You were right. Her art is different but it's very, very good." I went on to say that Stacy had threatened to throw the painting away. In the weeks since she painted it, her visual tracking had improved. Once she saw the blank side of the canvas, she was embarrassed by it—it was a painful reminder of her disabilities. Leah said, "Don't you dare let her throw this out! Do you realize how magnificent this is? Mona, this is truly miraculous!"

In May, we severed our relationship with the speech therapist at the hospital. We'd been unsuccessful in bridging the gap between her techniques and Stacy's needs. Stacy completed another one credit hour independent study with Donna Brown. She had been thinking a lot about whether she wanted to complete the art teacher education program she was majoring in. She worried about the rigors of classroom teaching and her ability, or inability, to maintain the required pace. We met with the head of the art department who supported Stacy's decision to switch her major to general art. They planned a class schedule for the upcoming fall semester. Stacy was still on track although she was moving slightly slower than she had before.

June brought Stacy's 23rd birthday and Patty's wedding. We flew to Houston. On the day of the wedding we darted back and forth through pouring rain frantically trying to keep everything dry. The storm clouds parted about half an hour before the ceremony. Dressed in flattering red dresses of their own choosing, Jeannie served as the maid of honor with Camy and Stacy as bridesmaids. Stacy wore red Crocs instead of heels but no one could tell. Jordyn was a junior bridesmaid. She was, after all, approaching her 10th birthday and was much too grown up to be a flower girl. When it came time for Stacy to walk down the aisle on the arm of her attendant, there wasn't a dry eye in the church. Patty made a beautiful bride—stunning in her strapless gown. I proudly escorted her to meet her new husband. It was impossible to find the right words to describe the love, pride, respect, and admiration that I felt for my incredible daughters.

We returned home and spent July and August preparing Stacy for her upcoming semester and the fulfillment of another one of her goals: driving. We worked with an out-patient rehabilitation center in Fort Collins. Stacy completed their driver education program and applied for an updated Wyoming license. Since hers had never been suspended, it was a simple procedure. Her little green Jeep had rested in my garage for over a year. There was no way she could safely get in and out of it let alone use the stick shift. We researched over fifty vehicles before we found one with the features she needed. We traded the Jeep for a Honda CRV. She was sad to sell it but thrilled with her renewed sense of freedom.

We were thrilled to receive a letter informing Stacy she had been selected as a recipient of the Hahn Alumni Scholarship from Craig Hospital. The financial assistance was greatly appreciated and came at just the right time.

Shortly before the semester began we met with the university's Disability Support Services (UDSS) coordinator Chris Primus to outline a plan for any accommodations Stacy might need in her courses: additional time for taking exams, use of a tutor or note taker, and books on audio tape. She was excited to work with Stacy. The assistance was provided cordially and respectfully. What a breath of fresh air!

We solicited the services of the Speech-Language and Hearing Clinic on campus to fill the gap in speech therapy. Lynda Coyle, the clinical director who mentors graduate student clinicians in the fields of audiology and speech for the Division of Communication Disorders, was thrilled to have Stacy as a client. The down side of working with the clinic was that Medicaid would not pay for the services because they were not in a hospital setting. Lynda helped us negotiate a fee we could live with. She desperately wanted her clinical students to work with Stacy. As a young stroke survivor, she was a unique specimen that most students do not have the opportunity to learn from. Stacy's agreement to participate in this way opened doors for her that we did not anticipate nor reap rewards from until much later. At that time, we were just pleased to be back in a setting that provided Stacy with reading and writing practice and classroom learning strategies.

Maintaining Stacy's Medicaid and Social Security coverage was a never ending battle. I could fill a stadium with the paperwork I've completed on her behalf. It seemed we'd finally find a representative who was conscientious and helpful only to lose them. During one particularly frustrating phone conference with Social Security, I questioned their reluctance to accept the decision made by Stacy's doctors that many of her disabilities were permanent. I asked what the issue was and how I could help. The man said "We do not believe Stacy is disabled therefore she does not meet the requirements for SSI and Medicaid benefits." We desperately needed to maintain those services so Stacy could continue having medical coverage. I suggested he come to Laramie and spend one hour with Stacy so he could see for himself what she was dealing with. He informed me, "Social Security does not do that!" I concluded, "Then tell me what we need to do to convince you!" He said many people stopped "pushing it" at this point and just accepted the decision. I told him that was not an option for us. Finally he said he would review her case with his supervisor. I thanked him for reconsidering. Three days later a letter arrived confirming her benefits would continue for one more year.

Stacy's decision to complete her degree meant making adjustments. She first finished the requirements for her incomplete printmaking course from the previous academic year. She came up with a new approach to asking for assistance. She hated asking for help so she'd simply say, "Mom, can I borrow your hands?" It was difficult for her to carve the bold Japanese design she had chosen into the wooden blocks she had to use with only one working hand, so I held them in place for her. She spent hours with her carving tools hunched over the blocks until she was comfortable with the finished product. I spent hours assisting her. She applied the ink and ran the prints. They came out beautifully and are some of my favorites. The X grade for the incomplete was removed and she received a B for the course.

Her second fall course was Life Drawing. She was back in the studio. She had to work twice as hard as she had before. Nothing came together the way she envisioned it. She was easily distracted because of her damaged frontal lobe. While she worked on one piece, she immediately thought of an idea for another one. The attention deficit was driving her nuts. Impulsivity was another issue intertwined with the first. She'd lay awake conceiving elaborate ideas for everything from paintings and sketches to reorganizing her movies and cds. She'd draw plans for bookshelves, sculptures, and a hundred different small art projects. Other times she'd crash and sleep for twelve hours straight. We had to do something. Dr. Shafer prescribed Provigil—a medication to help with her attention. It improved her focus tremendously.

Stacy really enjoyed her course and the time in the studio with other students. One day as she was entering the Fine Arts building, she struggled to carry all her supplies for class that day. She stopped a female student and asked for help. The girl retorted, "What, your arm's broke?" Stacy replied, "No, I had a stroke." The girl asked, "Just now?" Stacy explained the whole story and eventually the girl carried the supplies for her. When Stacy told me about the incident, my first instinct was to track down the girl and shake her until her teeth rattled. Stacy insisted I do no such thing. She admitted it was humiliating and that she had fought the urge to cry but she reminded me, "What doesn't kill me makes me stronger, Mom." *Yes, I thought, but just how strong does she need to be?*

For her final class project in Life Drawing, Stacy had to complete a self portrait. The instructions called for something that captured the artist in a setting or pose that others would not expect. She planned carefully for what she wanted to capture. She asked for my help. I ran the digital camera while she posed for some dramatic shots. Head bowed, arms clasping her bare knees, she tenderly cradled her own naked body. Using the photos as her guide, she began the life-sized charcoal sketch. We taped a huge piece of heavy paper to one large open wall in our living room. With intricate precision she drew herself—fragile, vulnerable, and sad. She titled the piece *Broken*. As she worked we often left the drapes open for additional light and shadow. Many times while she was absorbed in drawing, we saw cars slow down as they passed on the street outside. Wanting to know what was so interesting to the passersby, Stacy went into the yard and stood gazing through the window from curb. From that distance, you could not see where the wall ended and the paper began. Her fantastic sketch resembled a striking mural.

We proceeded through fall and were thrilled when Patty called to say she and Kevin were expecting. The baby was due the following May. She was ecstatic and sick. They traveled to Laramie for Thanksgiving. She was miserable with morning sickness. The weather was horrible. A few days later, Stacy finished her class and received a C. She was happy with the grade and the experience.

Jeannie joined us for Christmas and we spent time in the mountains hiking on easy trails so Stacy could enjoy the winter wonderland. We were disappointed that Stacy's friends had gradually distanced themselves from her until she had no one except her sisters and me. She treasured her time with Jeannie. Their special bond was not diminished by the distance between them.

Stacy had been dreaming of being able to wear her beloved cowboy boots again so for Christmas I planned to give her a new pair. I took her to the western wear store so we could make sure of the size and fit first. She worried that her stubborn left foot wouldn't cooperate. When she successfully slid her foot into the boot, her eyes widened, and the astonished look on her face was priceless. *Yes!* I had tears in my eyes. I know it was such a simple little thing but it felt huge to me. We ended 2004 quietly and looked forward to 2005.

Chapter Seventeen

Rough Terrain

We will either find a way, or make one!

~Hannibal~

From the beginning of our journey, I kept record of our progress on a daily basis for in the beginning each moment was fragile thus handled with care. Another new year found us in the throes of real life—existence *after* the traumatic event—no longer in the midst of it. It is painfully true that life goes on which is exactly what it did for us. My journal writing slowed a bit from daily to weekly entries.

Stacy enrolled in another course in spring 2005. It was one of her required history courses and she struggled to stay focused. She developed a fascination with facial reconstruction and forensic art. She spoke with some FBI field representatives at a criminal justice conference on campus. One encouraged her to pursue the possibility. Sketching was something she *could* do with one hand.

Laramie is home to two well known professionals in this area: nationally recognized forensic artist Sharon Long and anthropology professor George W. Gill, an expert in the field of racial identification. Stacy met with Professor Gill who encouraged her to take an anthropology course to see what she thought of the subject matter. Her contact with Ms. Long was by phone and also pointed her toward coursework first. She spoke with her adviser and decided to take an anthropology course in the fall.

In February, after weeks of suspicion and heartbreak, Patty called to say her new husband had changed his mind about marriage and parenthood. He left her for another woman and a less cluttered life. She was devastated, angry, hurt, and six months pregnant. I was furious and desperately wanted to dismember the man *slowly*. I hadn't felt that kind of anger since Camy's divorce. Stacy, Jeannie and Camy were heartbroken for their sister and felt helpless. You know, it's a nasty job being a woman sometimes!

I couldn't run to Patty's side the way I wanted to and she couldn't come home to Laramie. She had a great job with medical benefits she desperately needed and was surrounded by loyal friends. Jeannie and Patty's friend Tina Krolczyk stepped in as labor and delivery coaches. We all anxiously awaited the birth of Patty's child—a daughter she planned to name Ellison Tate. Jordyn was thrilled at the prospect of having a cousin.

In early April, as we anticipated ways of celebrating Stacy's two year survival mark, we had a scare that shook us to the core. One night Stacy's little dog Harley startled me from a sound sleep with a frantic bark. I stumbled to follow him down the hall to Stacy's room. I found her on the floor, tangled in her blankets, unresponsive. It took some effort to remove the twisted covers. She finally roused but couldn't stand and had no idea how she came to be in a heap on the floor. She was confused and had difficulty speaking. Before I could react she vomited all over herself, me, and the blankets. What an overwhelming feeling of déjà vu!

I lifted Stacy onto her bed and helped her dress in clean sweatpants and a t-shirt. I put a heavy sweatshirt on her and stretched her out on the bed. I ran to my room, threw on some clothes, grabbed my purse and cell phone, and prepared to leave the house. I tucked little Harley into a warm blanket on the couch and called Camy to tell her what happened. Exactly as I had done that April day two years before, I pulled my car onto the front lawn and helped Stacy into the front seat. I was taking no chances this time. I headed out of Laramie to Cheyenne.

I could not believe we were there in the Cheyenne medical center again. It was just too weird to comprehend. Stacy was ushered inside and taken to CT immediately. Dr. Shafer was out of town—due back in three days. Another neurologist was called. He wanted to do a MRI but needed to know if it was a permitted procedure with Stacy's shunt. I gave him all the information I had about doctors, procedures, etc. He called Swedish Hospital in Denver and they faxed everything he needed. The MRI was done—much to my relief.

When the results came in, we were so glad to know Stacy had not suffered another stroke but concerned that they suspected a seizure. It was almost two years to the day since her stroke. Most seizure disorders in stroke survivors develop before that much time has elapsed. I had hoped we could avoid this and truly thought we were in the clear. We scheduled a follow-up appointment with Dr. Shafer—the first on his schedule for the day he returned from his annual vacation. Stacy was scared about what a seizure disorder might mean. I worried about it too and know I aged significantly as a result of the frightening experience.

A seizure is best described as sudden abnormal electrical activity in the brain. Traumatic brain injury increases the likelihood of seizures. After a stroke, the healing brain tissue is easily excited and acts differently than it did before. Sometimes the damaged neurons just freak out. Let's say for one minute that the overly excited neurons are three-year-olds who haven't napped in four days and have eaten too many sugary snacks. Imagine if you can, a few million of them all running in different directions, shrieking, bumping into one another, and generally wreaking havoc on everything in sight. That is my analogy of a seizure.

Dr. Shafer ordered an electroencephalogram (EEG) and other lab work. The results supported his suspicion. Stacy had a slight seizure disorder but it could easily be controlled with medication. He explained that the scar tissue in Stacy's brain could not perform the way her other brain tissue did. It was a scary experience but she came through it without much residual damage. She went back to class and finished her history course. It was difficult for her to concentrate but she did her best. This time she received a D but didn't challenge the grade. She was glad she hadn't failed and that the class was over. She planned to rest and prepared to do better in the fall.

On May 19, Patty's obstetrician induced labor. The following morning she gave birth to a healthy baby girl. Jeannie and Tina were with her through every minute of labor and delivery. Stacy and I left Laramie and drove the 1,200 miles to Houston through Colorado, New Mexico, and Texas. We decided to drive instead of flying so we could have more flexibility with our schedule. We stayed for three weeks.

Stacy was afraid to hold little Ellie for fear she'd drop her but she did great. She'd cuddle the baby close and tell her stories about everything she could think of. A precious darling with dark eyes and darker hair, Ellie would stare at Stacy's face, her tiny mouth pursed into an "o," and listen to her voice with a serious look on her face. I soaked up every second knowing there was no way I could stay. We celebrated Stacy's 24th birthday with Patty, Jeannie, and Ellie. As much as we hated to leave, I had to return to work. We prepared everything we could think of for Patty's new role as a single mom. Jeannie gave up her apartment and moved in with Patty. We all cried the morning we left Houston.

Stacy enrolled for the fall semester—six credit hours of Cultural Anthropology and the History of North American Indians. With continued financial support from scholarships and Pell grants, she was set for the academic year. Before classes started, we met again with Dr. Sobel, her orthopedic surgeon. The first three toes on Stacy's left foot had gradually curled under making it difficult to walk. Another procedure was scheduled. The toe joints were surgically broken and reset with metal pins to hold them in place. Casted again, she started the fall semester with pins sticking out of the ends of her toes. Several times she bumped her foot while going up and down the stairs to her history class. It was held in a building without an elevator. She remarked that she felt a jolt of pain all the way to her shoulders and had to stop to catch her breath. When the pins were finally removed, she kept them as souvenirs! She worked diligently all semester and finished with two Cs.

That fall, Stacy was fortunate to meet two Wyoming artists that she greatly admired. Dave McGary, a native of Cody, Wyoming is a nationally acclaimed realism sculptor—capturing Native Americans in amazing lifelike detail. In September he attended the unveiling and dedication ceremony on our university campus for his sculpture of Shoshone Chief Washakie called *The Battle of Two Hearts*. Stacy, Jordyn, and I sat in a crowd of students, administrators, government officials, descendants of the chief, and members of the Shoshone tribe. Afterward Stacy met and visited with Mr. McGary. He encouraged her to never give up on her dream of being an artist.

Western portrait artist Carrie Ballantyne captures her subjects—the men, women and children of Wyoming and surrounding area ranches—in much the same way as her mentor James Bama. Stacy had been fascinated by her technique since she first saw her work on the cover of a western art magazine. We knew Ms. Ballantyne had a home in Sheridan, Wyoming and attended the same church as my brother Arlin. She had photographed my dad as a potential subject, so Mom asked if she would be willing to visit with Stacy. When we went to Sheridan to be with our family there for Thanksgiving that fall, Carrie invited us to her home and talked with Stacy at length about sketching different facial features one at a time until she had mastered each. She presented Stacy with a signed print, a warm hug, and her optimistic opinion that Stacy should embrace her art once more.

On December 22, Stacy reached a significant milestone—she "graduated" from physical therapy. We had a little party in the therapy gym at the hospital. She had worked so hard to gain every possible use of her arm and leg. Once she reached the current plateau, the therapists could no longer justify the need for continued therapy to Medicaid. We'd have to continue on our own.

Patty's divorce had been finalized in November so she and Ellie came to Wyoming for Christmas. We hadn't seen them since May. Ellie was now six months old and so much fun. She would cuddle close to Stacy on the couch and listen intently to stories. We took her to the mountains and played in the snow. She'd squeal with delight and made everyone laugh. I rocked her to sleep and held her close. I hated to take them to the airport for their return flight. I knew it would be at least six more months before we saw them again.

We closed out another year with a sense of accomplishment and pride in our family resiliency. Saying goodbye to 2005 meant reflecting on all that had happened during the previous twelve months. What a year of ups and downs! I was counting on 2006 to be a better year for all of us. We needed one!

Chapter Eighteen

Billboards

*Every artist dips his brush in his own soul, and paints his own
nature into his pictures.*

~Henry Ward Beecher~

Pablo Picasso said, "Painting is just another way of keeping a diary." Stacy's recovery and acceptance of what she could not change came, in large part, through her art. She chronicled her own journey without being aware that she was doing so. As I watched her at work in her studio—setting out all her tools, mixing paint, preparing her brushes and palette—it was hard to believe that the part of her brain that held her artistic expression and ability to conceive the complex thought processes necessary to plan and carry through with an idea had been so severely compromised.

Spring 2006 found Stacy back in the studio at the university. She enrolled in six credit hours of required painting classes. As the semester progressed her painting evolved and she began putting a few of her pieces together for a series—a class requirement. The subject of each was a separate part of her recovery: first memories, therapy, adapting to her disabilities. She and I talked about adding some work from before her stroke and forming a collection. She chose a title for the grouping, *A Piece of My Mind*. That April, in celebration of three years of stroke survival, Stacy invited family and friends to view the collection. We rented a downtown building used for special occasions, made some snacks and punch, and opened the door on her first exhibit.

Stacy authored the program and wrote the descriptions of each piece. The introduction read as follows:

Life can change in the blink of an eye. I know that all too well. On April 10, 2003, at the ripe old age of 21, I suffered a massive stroke. After three brain surgeries, months of hospitalization and rehabilitation, I returned home to a life much different than the one I had known. Prior to my stroke I was an art education major in my junior year at the University of Wyoming. I have changed my educational focus a little but art is still a huge part of my life. It has always been an outlet for me but now it offers healing powers. Through my art, I am able to convey feelings that are difficult to describe in mere words. "A Piece of My Mind" is a special collection of works, in a variety of mediums that hold great significance to me and my life. The theme of the collection is actually two-fold. First, the title represents the literal loss of the part of my brain that was damaged. Known for being outspoken before my stroke, I have jokingly remarked since that I can no longer give someone a piece of my mind because I cannot afford to lose any more than I already have! Secondly, the collection is my way of expressing something very painful, personal and profound. No one can know what a stroke feels like or what it does to a body unless they experience it for themselves. This collection is meant to convey some of those feelings. Three years later, I am ready to share this work with you. I hope you will view each piece of my collection with an open mind and receptive heart.

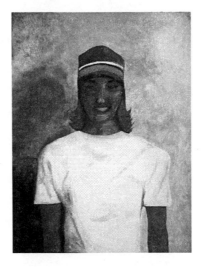

Me
November 2002

Painted before my stroke, this self portrait is the old me. The first Stacy loved to snowboard, ride my bike, rollerblade, and drive my Jeep. I loved horses and being outside doing anything with them. The world and my future, as I thought it would be, lay before me. I was carefree and silly sometimes. Never in a million years would I have imagined my life would change so drastically in such a short time.

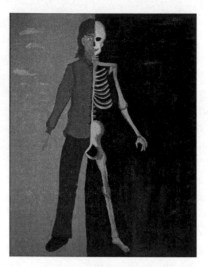

April 10
February 2006

This painting represents what happened to me the day of my stroke. My left side, as I knew it, died. My body and my life were torn in half. The right side, my semi-conscious self, fought to hold onto life. The "dark side" nearly pulled me under.

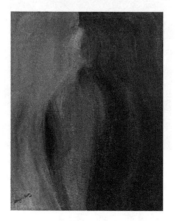

Bound
February 2006

My first conscious memories after my stroke are of being unable to move. I was also unable to speak. I knew something was wrong with my body but I did not know what was holding me down. It was similar to being bound like a mummy.

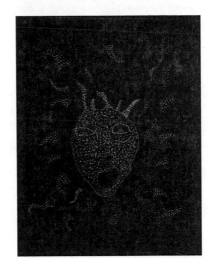

Scream
February 2006

Stroke doesn't care what you had planned for tomorrow or next week. It takes your spirit and destroys everything that was normal in your life. If you let it, it will dissolve everything that was "you." No matter how many times you scream and cry, you cannot hit it back the way you want to. You cannot make it hurt the way it has hurt you. You suffer in silence, screaming inside, not knowing how to make your pain go away.

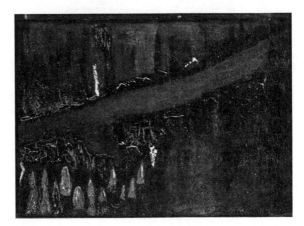

Tortured
March 2006

In therapy the pain is torture. It draws you into a unique hell. Deeper and deeper you go because it hurts so bad and you don't want to hurt anymore. You just want the pain to go away. At some point you need to stop and move toward another path. One that takes you out of the hell.

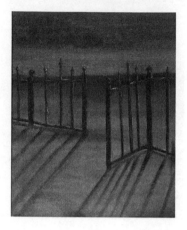

Grief
February 2002

Painted before my stroke, this piece took on new meaning. One of my class assignments was to draw a piece of paper from a hat that had an emotion written on it. Then I had to "illustrate" that emotion using a random color also drawn from a hat. Grief busts into your life. It throws open the gate that secures your life and with reckless abandon floods your soul with pain and sorrow.

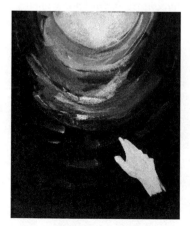

Decision
February 2006

There comes a point when you can decide to reach out, even when you are not sure what is out there waiting for you or how you will feel when you come out of the dark place where you have been. It is a decision you have to make for yourself when you are ready for the journey.

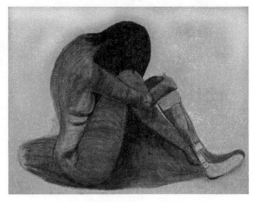

Broken
November 2004

This piece is a life-sized self portrait. It was a class assignment for Life Drawing, my first studio class after my stroke. It was difficult for me to return to school and allow myself to "feel" my work again. I wasn't sure if I could draw anymore.

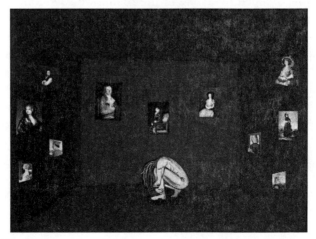

On Display
February 2006

Having a disability can isolate you from the world because people tend to stare and assume rather than attempt to understand. This piece portrays the feelings I have of being the same on the inside while appearing somewhat different on the outside.

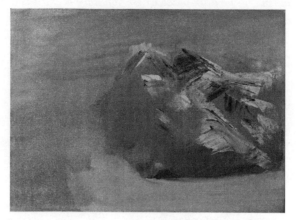

Untitled

My first attempt at painting after my stroke. I have always loved painting landscapes. I particularly love the mountains. As I painted this I was unaware that I used only half of the canvas. The damage to my brain left me with a left-side deficit that impacted my ability to visually track to the left.

The exhibit touched everyone in the room. We saw familiar faces while others were noticeably absent. Standing in the back of the room, much to our surprise, was Dr. Sobel. He had called us a few days before the show to say he would not be able to attend but appreciated being invited. When I saw him, I mentioned that I was glad he had changed his mind. He was so moved and incredibly pleased that he had chosen to bring his wife and son along. He hugged Stacy warmly and congratulated her on a job well done.

Stacy asked her guests to autograph a special paint pallet she had prepared with a silver metallic finish and to add their comments to her guest book. Some of the comments are as follows:

Dear Stacy—I really liked your work. I think it was great. Keep it up! Love, Jordyn

Thank you for sharing your life-journey with us through your talent and your words. May God bless you on your upward journey.

Thank you, Stacy, for the opportunity to see a small bit of your experience. There's so much of your spirit's desire to grow that we can never know. You are amazing!

Stacy—What an incredible exhibit! You have managed to express yourself so well through your art but also through your written and verbal descriptions. Way to go! Donna Brown

Dear Stacy—I don't have words. Thank you for inviting me to your wonderful showing!! I can't express how moving and special it was. You are truly an extraordinary woman! It has been a privilege to know and work with you. Thank you for allowing me to accompany you on part of your journey. Sincerely, Frances Price

Your experience has been of great inspiration to me personally. When I first saw you, a broken child after your stroke, I never thought to see you whole again. Yes, I know, there is something gone, but there is something added too. It is a precious gift.

Stacy was overwhelmed by the response to her one-woman-show. Many people made offers to purchase individual paintings but Stacy felt they should not be separated—their power came from the story told by all the pieces together. Lynda Coyle, her speech coordinator was particularly inspired by the experience. She suggested to her supervisor that the university's College of Health Sciences consider buying the entire collection. After a few weeks of negotiation, Stacy agreed to sell it. What an accomplishment for someone who was told they would never be an artist again!

Chapter Nineteen

Coasting

Perseverance is not a long race; it is many short
races one after another.

~Walter Elliott~

Success can be measured so many ways. In my opinion, our society often forgets that the winner of a race is not the only important participant. I remember a televised interview with Olympic figure skater Michelle Kwan after a silver medal was awarded to her. The reporter kept going on and on about how she "lost the gold" to another competitor. Finally Ms. Kwan stopped him and said, "I *won* the silver!"

That spring semester ended and, to Stacy's astonishment, she earned an A and a B which placed her on the Vice President's honor roll. An official letter congratulating Stacy came from Academic Affairs. We sent an e-mail thank you and said how much the acknowledgement meant to both of us. The vice president wrote back and asked Stacy if she would consider having a story written about her stroke and return to the university for the campus magazine. She agreed. We met with the editor who suggested Stacy write the story herself. No one else could tell it better. A university photographer came to our house and captured Stacy at work in her studio. Images of her collection mingled with her words for a four page spread that was scheduled to appear in the winter edition of *UWYO*. The following are some passages from the original unedited version of the article she submitted:

My first conscious memory in the hospital was of waking and
feeling as if I was wrapped like a mummy. I couldn't move. I couldn't

speak because I had a breathing tube. My entire family was at my bedside and I was confused as to why they were there. They were relieved to know I could see and recognize them. When Dr. Shafer asked me to move a finger, I thought it was silly that everyone was so excited about such an ordinary thing. I didn't understand the significance of my ability to comply with that simple request. Everything was foggy and I drifted in and out. I vaguely remember Mom telling me that my left side was paralyzed.

I became more aware of my surroundings. I remember seeing myself in the mirror for the first time and not recognizing myself. My eyes were black and blue from the surgery. I was so pale. My bald head was wrapped with bandages. I had a screen above my bed that featured rotating photos of scenic places. At times I would catch my reflection in the glass and think "that's what a dead person looks like." When the bandages were removed I resembled Frankenstein. My head was horribly out of proportion. I had a huge lump on my forehead from a buildup of brain fluid under my scalp. It was like a science fiction movie. I was sure this couldn't be real. I wanted to scream that I was trapped inside someone else's body. "I am Stacy! I am not this person! Someone, please help me get out of this body! God, please!"

Nights were long and scary. Mom would leave the hospital for a few hours of sleep. I would lie awake anxiously waiting for her to come back. It took forever for morning to come. I begged her to just take me home. I didn't want to be in the hospital anymore. I insisted she could care for me, and promised I wouldn't be a burden. With tears in her eyes, she refused. She said we both needed to learn how to deal with my disability. I was angry and hurt. At the time I didn't realize the strength it took for her not to give in. Now I can honestly say I am glad she didn't listen to me.

In therapy we set goals and measured success by each milestone I reached. I practiced walking a little further each day. I worked on my organizational and social interaction skills—impulsiveness and attention deficit are effects of the frontal lobe damage to my brain. I struggled with my inability to visually track to the left. I did not realize that when I wrote all my words were scrunched onto the right margin of my paper. If I ever hoped to drive again I would need to overcome this obstacle. In the middle of these challenges, I decided to return to school.

People have asked me if I would go back and change things if I could. There is no answer to that question. No one has the opportunity to change the past, but we do have the power to make our own future.

Mom told me early on that anyone can give up; it requires no effort at all. It's fighting back that's hard, that is where true courage lies. I am just stubborn enough to believe that. I think it's in my genes.

If I can give any advice from my experience, it would be to never take a single thing for granted. If someone you know has a serious accident or illness, ask yourself how you would want to be treated if you were in their shoes. Try to recognize how much they want and need your friendship. If you have difficulty accepting the changes in them, try to imagine how they feel. Never let an argument or disagreement go unresolved. Tell the people in your life how much they mean to you. Do not miss an opportunity to laugh. Treasure the small things in life and don't worry about the things you have no control over. Finally, take a serious look at how you measure your failures and your successes.

I have regained basic shoulder and elbow movement, but haven't mastered fine motor skills in my hand. I battle fatigue daily. I continue to make progress, but brain tissue takes 10 times longer to heal than any other part of the body. I remain hopeful.

My life is taking me in directions I didn't anticipate. When my family waited and wondered about the extent of the damage to my brain, they were told I would probably never be the artist I was. In some respects the doctors were right: I am a better one.

Before the magazine hit the presses, Stacy heard through mutual friends that her former teacher, Leah Griffin, had been diagnosed with ALS—better known as Lou Gehrig's disease. Stacy was devastated and saddened by the news. She had been out of touch with Leah for several months but assumed it could be easily explained because they both were often busy. She wanted to show her love and support any way she could. She also wanted to know more about the disease that had struck her dear friend. I helped her do some research. ALS is a progressively degenerative disease for which there is no cure. It attacks the motor neurons in the brains. Eventually all control of muscle movement is lost and the person is paralyzed. Stacy cried for Leah and for the fact that she could do nothing to stop this horrible disease. She told me she thought she understood how I felt when I couldn't stop her stroke.

In May, little Ellie celebrated her first birthday. Patty finished the school year with her first graders and prepared to teach a few weeks of summer school for extra pay. In late June, she and Ellie arrived in Laramie for a month of vacation. Stacy and I traveled with them to Sheridan for the Cooper family reunion. Camy was absent because Jordyn had to have her appendix removed a few weeks earlier. Seasonal retail commitments kept Jeannie in Texas. My siblings have tried to organize the event every four years. The 2006 gathering was held in the Big Horn Mountains at a camp ground that provided the perfect setting. My parents embraced each member of their huge extended brood. This occasion was particularly special for them because they had welcomed five new great-grandchildren (Ellie was one!) the previous year. They referred to them as "The Five in 2005"–three girls and two boys. We spent four days in the bosom of our family and loved every minute of it. Those who had not seen Stacy since her stroke were amazed at her progress.

Prior to leaving for the family reunion, Stacy and I completed modifications of a recumbent bicycle that my brother Arlin helped us purchase. Stacy researched several models and finally settled on one from KMX Karts. A local bike shop assembled it for her and removed the left handle. Technically a low-profile tricycle with two small wheels in front and one larger wheel in the back, Stacy could shift and turn using only the right hand levers. On straight stretches, she often pedaled with only her left leg. It gave her a new form of exercise and considerably strengthened her weaker leg.

In October, Stacy and I were invited to participate in a professional conference on campus titled "The Many Faces of Stroke." The focus of the conference was a discussion of rehabilitation, recovery, and re-entry for stroke survivors of all ages. The keynote speaker, Dr. Dale Strasser, an associate professor and physician at Emory University of Medicine in Georgia, talked about rehabilitation teams. Stacy agreed to serve on the panel that gave their opinions of his approach. After listening to the keynote, I was squirming in my seat. He talked about teams of therapists, nurses, doctors, and various specialists but forgot one important component: the patient's family.

When it was Stacy's turn to speak, she brought up that subject. When it came time for comments from the audience, I stood and grilled the speaker with a barrage of questions. He was clearly dumbfounded by my implication that he was missing the mark by a mile. He even went so far as to say family members interfered and were too emotionally involved. I asked what he thought they should do instead—after all they *were* enmeshed in the situation—physically, emotionally, and spiritually. They knew the patient better than anyone else on the "team." What did he expect of them? After the team of professionals disbanded, who did he think picked up the slack and carried on? Others in the room supported my point of view but I clearly upset Dr. Strasser more than I intended to. I owe him an apology for reacting so passionately. I hope he understands how near and dear the subject is to me.

Over lunch with the conference participants, Stacy gave a slide presentation of her collection and talked about her stroke and return to college. She spoke candidly and answered questions from the audience which was comprised primarily of college students her age. Afterward, Dr. Strasser posed for publicity photos with her, shook her hand, and joined the rest of the attendees in watching as the collection was unveiled—beautifully framed and ready to be permanently displayed. The *Stacy Gupton Collection* found a new home on the second floor of the Health Sciences building.

In addition to the conference, Stacy completed two courses in the fall semester. Still interested in forensic art, she had enrolled in a criminology course. The other was her final English requirement. She struggled with the volume of required readings in Criminology and completed the course with a D. She wrote often and well in her English class because she connected with the professor and several of her classmates. She finished that course with a B.

The full color *UWYO* magazine came out just before finals week. Stacy's piece *Decision* graced the front cover. We sent copies to everyone we knew. The article received rave reviews. Our friend Treva sent a congratulatory email:

> *Hello you two! We got the magazine yesterday. It sent chills up my spine reading the article. Stacy, you did an excellent job. Your artwork featured was amazing!!!! When I was finished, I praised the Lord that you are still here and living a fulfilling life. You are a miracle, Stacy, and you have an amazing mom who loves you very much! You two are very special to me.*

What a way to end the semester and the year! We were kicking back, reflecting on Stacy's good fortune, and planning her next collection when the props came out from under us and we landed hard.

Chapter Twenty

Off Balance

We could never learn to be brave and patient if there
were only joy in the world.

~Helen Keller~

Life has a way of bringing you around full circle once you begin healing and recovery. You find yourself strolling along feeling like you can finally catch your breath and relax. You begin to enjoy some of the minor details that you hadn't had time to even think about. When you have concentrated day and night on staying alive or keeping someone else alive, little things go unnoticed—the sparkle of new snow, your breath visible on a cold morning, rosy pink cheeks on all the children passing by on their way to school. I think it is so important that life be lived and not held in limbo; however, sometimes the actions and choices of others slam into you and throw you off balance when you least expect it.

Late on the night of December 15, 2006, I had a phone call from my former brother-in-law, Neil's brother. Earlier that day, Neil crossed the center line of a remote highway in Utah causing a fiery head-on collision that claimed the lives of a lovely couple from Ogden. He had survived but was in a trauma center with burns, broken bones, and massive internal injuries. Our world turned upside down.

It was after midnight when the call came in. Neil's brother gave me the number for the hospital in Utah. I sat for awhile trying to come to terms with this tragedy and come up with a plan for telling the girls. I was particularly worried about how Stacy would react.

I called the trauma center first. The nurse I spoke to was a saint. She explained Neil's horrific injuries. It was inconceivable that he had even lived through the accident. The situation was so precarious; she could not predict what the next few minutes would bring. She asked if she could be brutally honest with me. I said, "Of course." She said, "Don't come here and don't let your kids see their father this way." I asked who would be the designated person to make medical decisions. She said it could be a spouse, parent, sibling, or child. She asked about his family. I said his parents were gone and he wasn't married as far as I knew. That left my girls and two other people—his brother and sister. I silently prayed. *Dear God, please don't leave this mess up to my girls.* I thanked the trauma nurse and hung up the phone. I had to break the new to my girls.

I prayed for strength. How I wish I could have spared my children from having to hear what I had to tell them. My heart broke for them. I called Camy first. She was completely and utterly devastated. Stacy heard us talking and called to me from her bedroom. She was shocked, hurt, sad, and angry at the news. I crawled into her bed and held her. I didn't know what else to do. We had to call Patty and Jeannie.

All of us worried about Stacy because she had been close to her dad and had tried to maintain a relationship with him for as long as she could. We all knew how confused she had been when he walked away and never looked back. Stacy had some good memories from when she had spent time on the ranch with her dad long after her sisters had decided not to go there anymore. If her sisters and I could have shielded her from this we would have given anything to do so.

The girls talked throughout the night and early morning. Each of them tried to recall the last time they had seen or spoken to their dad. They tried to conjure positive memories but each one was linked to another unpleasant one that was tough to be reminded of. Stacy mentioned telling her dad to find his own ride that time when he called her from jail. Camy remembered the conversation she had with him about staying sober or staying away. For Patty it was the recollection of observing him from a distance when she was out dancing with some college friends and realizing he did not recognize her.

Jeannie talked about the time Neil showed up at the house, drunk and angry, when she was home alone. She had called me at work in a panic because she didn't know what else to do. I raced home to find him sitting in my rocking chair with his head in his hands. I escorted him out of the house. I knew from experience that trying to talk to him while he was drunk could be risky because he was often irrational. He staggered on the front lawn and told me he just wanted his old life back. Then he asked me an odd question, "So how'd we do?" Confused I asked what he meant. He continued talking, his words thick and slurred, "As parents? How'd we do?" Looking him straight in the eye, my voice shaking with emotion, I answered, "*I* did a hell of a job." I turned my back on him, went back in the house, and called the police. They picked him up as he turned the corner at the end of our street and took him to jail.

A few days later I testified at Neil's hearing. I begged the judge to require some kind of counseling for alcohol abuse while had him in custody. I insisted, "Please do something—before he kills someone." When Neil was arrested after my call, he already had an outstanding warrant from another county so he had to serve a sentence there before he was returned to Laramie. He spent six months in our local jail. When he was released, he had called Stacy. We were sickened by what he had done. All of the memories that flooded our minds were from years before but none of us had anything more current or substantial to hold onto. The sad truth was my exact prediction had come true and it tore me up inside to think of the immeasurable loss.

Camy talked to the staff at the trauma center and agreed to fly to Salt Lake City. I would have gone in her place if I could have. Before she left, the four girls had come to a consensus—no heroic measures—but by the time Camy arrived in Utah, Neil's sister was already there. She assumed responsibility for all medical decisions taking it out of the girls' hands. I felt guilty that I was grateful for that. Neil's prognosis was . . . well, there really wasn't one. No one could believe he was still hanging on or that he would be able to for any significant length of time. Camy stayed three days and came home.

Patty and Ellie flew to Laramie for Christmas because they had already purchased their tickets. Jeannie couldn't get a reservation at the last minute or time off from work for more than one day so she stayed in Houston. We hated for her to be alone. On Christmas Eve we sat in church, holding hands, somber and sad on what should have been a joyous holiday. We said goodbye to the year that had held so much excitement and growth for Stacy, and such grief and pain for all of us.

Chapter Twenty-One

Taking a Detour

Patience and perseverance have a magical effect
before which difficulties disappear and obstacles vanish.

~John Quincy Adams~

According to the Department of Criminal Investigation, family members of people who commit horrific crimes often suffer in silence with feelings of anger, self-doubt, shame and guilt. They often are depressed and have trouble concentrating or sleeping. My girls were all dealing with the fallout from their dad's accident. Camy maintained contact with their aunt and provided all of us with daily updates. Stacy, Patty, and Jeannie decided not to go to see their dad. Their decision was not an easy one.

There comes a time in life when you realize your parents are just imperfect people like everyone else. My girls had never asked for perfection from their dad but they had dreamed of normalcy. More than anything, they mourned for what they wished they'd had—a childhood free of fear. Each of them tried to move forward and not dwell on it, but the situation 'sat' in our midst like a dead elephant that stank and no one had the power to dispose of. It was a mess and I hated it. They did not deserve this but there was nothing I could do. I was helpless.

Everyone went through the motions. They had responsibilities, jobs, children, and bills to pay. Stacy enrolled in two classes for spring semester; one oil painting class and an anthropology lecture. Being in the studio kept her mind occupied with more positive thoughts. She painted several pieces and genuinely enjoyed the students in her class. The anthropology course was challenging but she was intrigued by Dr. Gill. She met with her disability services advisor, Chris Primus and was introduced to another helper, Athena Kennedy, who would be her Student Success Services (SSS) advisor.

In March, Stacy and I were invited to Professor Virginia Vincenti's Family Decision Making class for a presentation on surviving a traumatic event via family support. The students were required to read Stacy's article. They were attentive and gracious—obviously inspired by what they read. The fact that Stacy was their same age made the topic more real to them. One student wrote this message afterward:

Hello Stacy,

Thank you very much for taking the time to share your experience with our class. You are one amazing woman! Your story made me cry. Your mother is also amazing! It sounds like she was there right by your side throughout the whole experience. What a wonderful mother and supportive family you have! I am so happy to hear of your recovery, and I wanted to tell you kudos for all the hard work you have had to endure during your recovery. You are quite the artist and a very good writer also! I wish you the very best life has to offer in your future endeavors.

Stacy reached a significant milestone that spring when she moved into her own apartment. In January, we had started the application process for federal housing assistance through a government sponsored program called Section 8. We found a two-bedroom bungalow that was perfect for Stacy. It had only two steps at the entrance and was within walking distance of campus. For me, the best part was that it was less than five minutes away from my house! Built in the 1960s, the apartment had a comfortable retro feel with brick work and wide windows. Stacy turned one bedroom into a studio.

Shortly after Stacy moved in we hosted a house warming party. Everyone was ecstatic about how much progress she had made. She settled in and made a strict schedule for herself. She did most of her own laundry, dishes, and other housework. I went over on weekends to help with any chores that were difficult for her to do alone. Have you ever tried to put a fitted sheet on a bed while using only one hand? Picture it in your mind—I would define that as instant craziness.

In April, as we neared the four year survival mark, Stacy mentioned that she was experiencing pain near her right ear. She thought maybe it was from a tooth. I began calling around to find a replacement for our dentist who had recently retired. I must have called twenty offices only to be told that they were not accepting new patients or did not accept Medicaid coverage. Before I could locate someone to work with her, Stacy suffered a grand mal seizure from the infection in her wisdom tooth and the resulting pressure that was too near her shunt.

That morning she came over to my house about 3:00 a.m. because the throbbing pain was so severe. She fell asleep for awhile but when she woke up she just wasn't herself. I called our new family doctor for some advice. He recommended taking Stacy to the hospital emergency room for some pain medication until I could get into a dentist. I had already made the decision to take her to anyone who could see her and worry about the financial part of it later. Camy happened to stop by my house and walked inside just as Stacy went into the seizure. I yelled at her to dial 911. Stacy was sitting in a chair—jaws clenched, her entire body jerking—and then she stopped breathing. We were frantic.

Camy and I were in a state of disbelief. We were reluctant to take Stacy to our local hospital but knew we had no choice. While I waited with Stacy in the ER, Camy called Dr. Shafer's office in Cheyenne to alert him. He was on vacation but due back the following day. The on-call neurologist assured us that as soon as Stacy stabilized, we could bring her there for follow-up.

Stacy was released from the hospital the same day with some pain medication for her tooth and a temporary increase in the dosage of her anti-seizure medication. She stayed at my house until we met with Dr. Shafer for a complete work up of blood tests. Her greatest fears were that she'd have to give up her apartment and her driving privileges but neither happened. Dr. Shafer adjusted the medication to a higher level and called his personal dentist who agreed to see Stacy. The impacted wisdom tooth was extracted—problem solved.

Stacy continued with her classes and passed with a D in her anthropology class and a C in painting. She was ready for summer and some down time. Patty and Ellie arrived in late June for a month of vacation with us. The girls rode a rollercoaster every day with their dad. Camy tried to maintain a civil relationship with her aunt so she could keep everyone else apprised of his condition.

In July, Camy made an impromptu visit to Utah. She said she just had an uncontrollable urge to go. She showed her dad photos and told him about each one of the girls. He couldn't speak but moved his lips in silent questions and comments that she struggled to decipher. Many of his 'words' were not easy for Camy. She had hoped for so much more. Disillusioned, she returned to Laramie with news of his deteriorating condition. She left the final decision up to her sisters but wanted them to know that their dad had never changed for the better. She did not encourage them go—she tried to spare them from what she had experienced. It reminded me of when they were kids and Camy tried to protect her little sisters from their dad's alcoholic rages. On August 18, Neil passed away. There was simply nothing more anyone could do for him. He was 51 years old.

Chapter Twenty-Two

The Home Stretch

If you want to get somewhere,
you have to know where you want to go and how to get there.
Then never, never, never give up.

~Norman Vincent Peale~

Grief is a natural emotion that a person must pass through when they lose someone. When the relationship you had with that person was an unhappy one, the sorrow and pain can be just as wretched as when the person was someone you loved dearly. I watched as my girls dealt with their dad's death. I did not know how they felt because my loving parents are still living so I tried not to be presumptuous and minimize their sorrow. My parents wrote to them.

> *Regardless of what anyone tells you, losing a parent hurts. You will always remember him with mixed feelings. Know that God understands. We love you, Grandpa and Grandma.*

The girls moved forward as they had so many times before. I was so proud of their strength and determination. I shook my head in admiration at the fantastic adults they had become. Camy met a wonderful man simply by chance and began dating after being single for almost eight years. We had never seen her so giddy and were so happy for her. The best part was that Jordyn was excited about it too. Jeannie was also in a serious relationship and made a switch to a new job. Patty moved to a new school in Houston and a new classroom where she would be teaching first grade.

Stacy enrolled in two courses for the fall, one in the studio and one to fulfill the first half of her foreign language requirement. The painting class was a piece of cake—she loved her time in the studio and created some striking pieces. Spanish, however, was not her friend. She struggled for weeks. The UDSS office hired a tutor for her. Even with constant coaching, it was impossible for her to retain the information. We tried different study techniques until her head swam. We met as a group—Stacy and me, her new advisor, Ricki Klages, and the UDSS/SSS staff. The recommendation was that Stacy should withdraw from the class rather than continue the impossible feat of mastering a new language. Everyone recognized the herculean effort she had made and assured her that lots of students withdraw from courses—some without good reason or half the effort she had put in. She hated the thought of giving up. Her academic and disability advisors worked with administrators in Arts and Sciences to obtain permission for Stacy to substitute two cultural content courses for the foreign language component of her art degree. It took some doing, but we finally convinced Stacy that she had not failed or given up—she had simply taken a different path.

October brought my fiftieth birthday and all the girls came together to celebrate it with me. It was wonderful. They showered me with gag gifts and decorated the house with black confetti and balloons. They insisted on taking me out to dinner. I was surprised when we entered the restaurant. Everyone from my office was there—the department head, the faculty, and the staff. Dinner was their gift to me and my family. I felt very appreciated and loved—and old!

I worked endlessly with Social Security to ensure continued coverage for Stacy. Sometimes I felt it was a futile effort but invariably it was worth it. Managing all her medications and doctor visits on my salary would have been impossible so we were thankful for the benefits she received. We were grateful when we heard Stacy was eligible for a slight increase in benefits because of her dad's death. We worked with Mike Allen again—he remembered us well. As before, he assured us the programs were intended for people like Stacy.

With only one course to concentrate on, Stacy finished the semester with a B in her painting class. The Christmas holiday was quiet although the weather was horrid. Patty and Ellie flew in for two weeks. Jeannie had to stay in Houston since she had come home for my birthday. We welcomed David Willems, known affectionately as Dave, Camy's significant other, into our big family of wild women. He didn't seem to mind. We closed out 2007 and welcomed 2008—a year we hoped would hold all good things.

Stacy and her advisor, Ricki Klages, met to outline her last remaining requirements for graduation. She chose one cultural course for spring semester—Chicano Folklore—and completed a replacement course for the art history she had withdrawn from the semester when she had her stroke. The course was offered online through one of Wyoming's community colleges. Although she was a bit apprehensive at first, having never taken an online class, it worked very well for Stacy. She finished the semester with an A in Chicano Folklore and a B in Art History. Since she did so well with her online class, she selected a second one for summer session to fulfill another history requirement.

The stroke survivors group from Cheyenne invited Stacy and I to one of their monthly meetings and asked us to talk about her recovery and her art. One thing about a stroke survivors group—there's always new members. That is just a fact of life with stroke. The group consisted of survivors and their spouses. Everyone was much older than Stacy but they treated her with respect and admiration. We felt welcome and appreciated. One person in the group was familiar to us—Robert Herb had attended the stroke conference with us and cheerfully admitted he had recommended we be invited. We enjoyed the meeting immensely and promised we would come back again.

Stacy and I marked five years of stroke survival by making a crazy quilt. She loved the idea and said it was an appropriate way to signify what she'd been through. Admittedly, we had sometimes been a little unhinged by her situation. We collected fabric for several months and used remnants from garments I made for the girls when they were younger. We had the best time sewing the colorful pieces together in a random pattern. Stacy and I had an agreement—she had to do some of the sewing. It wasn't easy for her to guide the fabric one-handed so some of the seams are uneven but that makes the quilt even more special. She remarked that it truly was a *crazy* quilt because it had nearly driven her over the edge while we made it. It was a labor of love that we enjoyed immensely.

Stacy had one of her regularly scheduled appointments with Dr. Shafer on the exact five-year anniversary—April 10, 2008. When we arrived at his office, we all went into the exam room where we first met. It was very emotional to be there and remember how terrified I had been that day. In some respects it felt like yesterday and in others like a lifetime ago. Stacy and Dr. Shafer talked like dear old friends about her classes and all the things she had been doing. I sat there counting my blessings and thanking God that we had found this man when we did. He was the reason we were all sitting there together. The significance of the day was not lost on him either. He remarked warmly, "Stacy, I am so glad you're here. It is always so good to see you."

When she was home during the holidays, Patty mentioned changes were being made in her school district. She was worried about the status of her job. In May, she and Ellie flew to Laramie for Mother's Day and interviews for local teaching positions. We drove to Sheridan to visit my parents and then took Patty and Ellie to the airport for their return flight. We waited to hear about the jobs. Within a few weeks, Patty was offered a first grade position in Laramie. She accepted, made arrangements to leave Texas after living there for 10 years, and began packing. In late June, she and Ellie came home to Wyoming.

Jeannie and her boyfriend Ryan Cheney helped with the cross-country move. Patty and Ellie unloaded their belongings at my little house while they looked for a place of their own. We spent the Fourth of July as a family enjoying the festivities that Laramie had to offer.

While we were in the park near my house for the annual celebration called "Freedom Has a Birthday," we saw Leah Griffin and her family. She was valiantly fighting ALS but was now confined to a wheelchair—unable to move other than to make slight nods of her head. Her spirit, however, was firmly intact as was her love for people. Leah talked with Stacy about how she continued to work with children and how accepting they were of her inability to physically show them how to complete an art project. She said, "Stacy, you don't need hands to teach—you just need the desire to teach." Afterward she sent Stacy this email message:

> *Dear Stacy,*
>
> *It was absolutely wonderful to see you in the park! Your smile is still contagious. I also enjoyed visiting with your mom. What is Patty looking forward to with her first graders? What are you doing in your Native American art class? Is it historical? What is your text? What kinds of questions, are, you asked?*
>
> *Please forgive spelling, typographical, and punctuation problems. I use a voice-activated system. So all kinds of things can occur. Some are indecipherable, some are silly, and most are frustrating. But it's a great way to keep in touch with people I care about—like you!*
>
> *Please describe your studio. What are you painting? What is your favorite color? What do you find the most challenging? Interesting? And important in your artwork? What classes do you have left in the fall? What will you wear to graduation? You must be very proud of your accomplishment.*
>
> *Smile.*
> *Love, Leah*

We spent a few relaxing weeks before Patty started her new job. Ellie started preschool and to our delight loved it! Stacy enrolled in seven credit hours and started her last semester without much fanfare. She met with her drawing instructor to make arrangements for one credit hour of independent study. She already knew the instructor from previous coursework but became reacquainted. They set a schedule to meet once a week. They planned an interesting semester of sketching together to strengthen Stacy's technique.

Women of the American West, a special Women's Studies offering that semester, intrigued Stacy so she chose it as her last cultural course. She wanted to be prepared so asked for the syllabus early, bought her books and began reading. It promised to be an exciting experience and one that could hold her attention.

The third class was a worry. It was Stacy's final art history requirement—19th Century European Art—intense subject matter. Stacy downloaded the syllabus and other course materials as soon as possible. She wanted to be ready. This would be her second encounter with her least favorite art history professor. The first had been in the spring semester of 2003 when Stacy had her stroke. She and the professor had some communication issues that Stacy had really struggled with. She had complained that it was her difficulties in that first class that had stressed her out so much during that semester. Many of her friends had jokingly teased her after her stroke about how "some people will do anything to get out of art history." Stacy admittedly had not done well in the course that semester but probably would have passed had she not been so rudely interrupted by a little thing called stroke.

Weekly sketches for Stacy's drawing class were fun. In her second course, trips to the library and museum archives in search of historical documents taught her about some of the incredible women who settled our state. She was never bored with these two courses. The art history course however was almost Stacy's undoing. She nearly walked away from everything she had worked so hard to achieve.

Stacy's relationship with her art history professor was strained from the first day of class. To keep her on track, she met at least once a week with her advisor and support team. A tutor was hired to help her with the mound of papers that had to be written. At mid-term Stacy faced the real possibility of failing and was frantic. Meetings were scheduled with the professor about the expectations for each assignment. The final was looming and Stacy was physically ill about the outcome. Her final essay—10 to 15 pages in length—had to present a unique perspective on the work of an artist from the period being studied. Stacy viewed the assignment with a mixture of horror and excitement. If all went well, this would be her last college assignment.

The topic of Stacy's final paper was a comparison of her own work with that of Spanish painter and printmaker Francisco Goya. It was a bold move and a leap of faith that she would be able to pull together enough evidence to show that his infamous Black Paintings—completed during a dark period of his life—were similar to some of the ones she had painted after her stroke. Rumored to have also had a stroke, Goya was often misunderstood. His style of painting took on a macabre feel and many felt he was suffering from dementia or insanity. Stacy thought otherwise. Her thesis statement supported one's basic need for expressing personal and painful life-changing events. Her stance was that sometimes life *is* dark and sometimes people *are* crazy but they have the right to paint their circumstances as *they* see them not as others want them portrayed. Life isn't always pretty and neither is art.

Every draft of the paper came back from the professor with negative comments. Stacy began to feel as though there was no chance of success and nearly resigned herself to failure. It was almost more than I could stand. She had come so far and I hated to see what this unfortunate encounter was doing to her.

As we neared the end of the semester, Camy provided a brief distraction for Stacy when she accepted Dave's marriage proposal. Forever a gentleman, he sought Jordyn's permission to ask for her mother's hand. The three of them began making plans for a summer wedding and a life together under one roof. I was thrilled for them—I had never seen Camy so happy and content. She and Jordyn deserved happiness and stability. Dave fit the role of husband and stepfather very well. It felt great to have my faith in men restored.

Commencement was upon us before we knew it. The university always holds their fall ceremony before final grades are posted. Stacy was afraid but decided to go through graduation as if she already knew she had passed all her classes. Art history be damned—she was going to participate in the ceremony. We gathered as a family—Stacy, Camy, Dave, Jordyn, Patty, Ellie, Jeannie, and me. The Arts and Sciences auditorium was crowded with faculty, administrators, and other families just like ours. The graduates in their brown and gold robes were hugging each other and having their pictures taken. It was bitterly cold for early December—the temperature outside hovered slightly above zero.

I helped Stacy find Ricki Klages, her advisor and department head. Each unit had a designated area where they met to prepare for the commencement march. Stacy and I met the day before with a member of the dean's staff for a private walk through. She was nervous but ready. Stacy and Ricki hugged warmly. She assured me she would be fine so I joined everyone inside and waited. Stacy reflected on the wait:

> Ricki and I talked while we were waiting. We decided we wouldn't worry about my art history grade. If for some reason I didn't pass, we would find an alternative class from another university and transfer the credits. I was going to cross that stage with my head held high and get my diploma. I was not going to worry about anything else.

The music began and the first department started the procession—Anthropology. The familiar strains of *Pomp and Circumstance* boomed in our ears. From my aisle seat I spotted them. Ricki carried the Art Department banner—more colorfully decorated than the others, it stood out. Right behind her was Stacy—wide smile and eyes twinkling. It took my breath away. My heart hurt from the sheer joy of the moment. She stopped by my seat and hugged me. She hugged Ellie too. She mouthed "I love you!" and continued down the aisle. Everyone had tears in their eyes.

All the graduating students and faculty were seated. The commencement speech was typical—long, dry, and uninspiring. We tried to stay focused but couldn't. We were there for Stacy. I crept closer to the stage for photos. She stood poised on the steps, ready to walk forward as soon as her name was called. When the dean read her name, we cheered. Ricki—first in line on stage—hugged her again. Stacy reached out and accepted the diploma from the dean's hand. She glanced at us and smiled. She recalled the moment:

> *I was so scared. When I had to come off the stage, I was afraid I would fall when I came down the stairs because there wasn't a railing on the right for me to hold onto. I stumbled but I caught myself before I fell. I saw some of my favorite professors waiting to congratulate me. Lots of people hugged me. Doug Russell handed me a bottle of bubbles. I tried to hold everything in my right hand. Mom was taking pictures. It felt so good!*

We spent the weekend enjoying each other's company and snapping photos. My favorite is one of Stacy and me together in our back yard. In accordance with graduation custom, the stole from the commencement regalia is supposed to be presented to someone who inspired and supported the graduate during their academic pursuit. Stacy gave hers to me. The photo caught us at that moment when she draped her yellow stole around my neck. What an honor!

Stacy hosted a small informal party at her apartment the afternoon after commencement. She wanted to thank everyone who had supported her while she was finishing her degree. My gift was a framed print of a jubilant little pig leaping off a dock into a beautiful lake. Titled *Kohler's Pig*—by Michael Sowa—the painting had been one of Stacy's favorites for several years. She had often remarked that she would love to experience such joyful abandon at some point in her life. I thought her graduation was the perfect time to present it to her.

My parents gave Stacy a Bible with all of their favorite verses highlighted. A gorgeous frame to display her diploma came from Camy, Patty, and Jeannie. Generous cash gifts would make it possible for her to purchase a new digital camera and supplies for her studio. One late arrival proved to be the gift worth waiting for. I had contacted Jean Milholland, Stacy's PT from Craig Hospital to update her on where we were and what we had been doing. She sent Stacy a necklace with the Craig emblem—a broken person on one side and a mended person on the other. Her note said:

> *Stacy—I am so proud of you and all you have done. This necklace is a reminder of how far you have come. You were broken when I met you but you have healed. You have accomplished so many things—you*

have much to be proud of. I look forward to seeing you and hearing about all that you are doing. Congratulations! Jean M.

While we were waiting *impatiently* for Stacy's grades to post, she met with Dr. Shafer for her six-month check-up. They chatted about graduation and he congratulated her on completing her degree. She talked with him about the grueling semester and the fact that she was holding her breath to see if she had actually passed art history. He was certain she had and told her so. She was her usual sassy self and gave him a bad time about not being in the audience the night of commencement. She had sent him an announcement but he had been forced to decline because of a previous commitment. He shook her hand professionally and then gave her a big warm hug. He said, "Stacy, I am so proud of you." She shrugged it off but smiled, her expression revealing her sense of accomplishment.

When we left the exam room, Stacy went first while Dr. Shafer and I walked side by side down the hallway behind her. He reached out and put his arm around my shoulder and said, "You know, Mona, if we had known then what we know now, maybe we wouldn't have worried quite so much." My eyes filled with tears. I thanked him and hugged him back.

Stacy was exhausted from the rigors of her last semester. On Tuesday, I took Jeannie back to the airport in Denver for her return flight to Houston. She hated to leave. Stacy's grades were due to be posted by noon on Thursday. Eight and half years came down to sweating over one final grade. Nothing appeared in her online student records until Friday morning. We checked each one: Independent Study—A, Women of the American West—C, and finally, 19th Century European Art—C. She had passed! Although she was not required to, she went to the Fine Arts Building to pick up her Goya paper. She really needed to know what her final grade had been. It was a B-. The hard work was over and her degree was official. Stacy had graduated with a 2.9 grade point average. Her race was finally won.

Chapter Twenty-Three

Reflection

When one door of happiness closes, another opens;
but often we look so long at the closed door
that we do not see the one that has been opened for us.

~Helen Keller~

I am amazed at how the human brain retains information. Memories stay with us often with incredible clarity. We sometimes associate a scent with a particularly fond childhood memory: chocolate chip cookies, spring wildflowers, or grandmother's perfume. Melancholy moments compel us to recall specific details such as what we were wearing or where we were standing when we heard a particular piece of news.

In 1963, I celebrated my sixth birthday a few short days before President John Fitzgerald Kennedy was assassinated. I recollect certain aspects of that day as if it were yesterday. I played quietly, sensing the drama even though I did not fully comprehend why my parents listened so intently to the radio. There have been other days and other events that have embedded themselves in my mind: the deaths of my baby sister and grandparents, my wedding, the births of my children, and the fire that destroyed my home the day after Thanksgiving in 1974. Human tragedies that touched the world also left their mark: the Challenger explosion, the Oklahoma City bombing, and September 11, 2001.

As I said before, I once thought people should have a warning of an impending life-altering event so they could brace themselves: a loud buzzer, a flashing neon sign, or a subtle tap on the shoulder—anything that would alert a person that something was about to drastically change. I once wanted a crystal ball so I could see the future and I once believed the myth that stroke happened only to older people.

I know now that if I had been able to see the future, I would have given my own life to change it. I can tell you that nothing can adequately prepare you for an accident or illness that leaves a loved one clinging to life, especially one who is young and full of energy and excitement about their future. I have learned more about stroke and traumatic brain injury than I would have imagined. I think I am a stronger person, a better mother, and a more understanding, compassionate human being because of the events of the past six and a half years. I believe I have grown. I was heartbroken, afraid, and angry, but I have been humbled and healed. I have been amazed, thrilled, proud, and astounded by the strength and perseverance of my own children. I am a fighter and will continue to fight until my last breath. I have a renewed sense of what's truly important in life.

In the final weeks of completing the manuscript for this book, I stayed in almost constant contact with our supporters by email and phone. I selected each chapter's quotation with a tremendous amount of thought and care. After I chose the one for this chapter, my sister-in-law Gena sent me another version that I want to share. "Whenever God closes one door, he always opens another, but sometimes it's hell in the hallway!" That is so true!

Looking back on Stacy's stroke, I realize that initially I was in a state of shock. I have never experienced such incapacitating fear or prolonged agony. I remarked earlier about the sensation of being frozen—my heart and lungs encased in a block of ice. Grief in its purest cruel form was eating me alive from the inside. My overwhelming disbelief kept me in a dream state. A desperate chant filled my mind like a silly song that sticks there after you hear it. Why? Why? Why?

When reality finally hit, it physically stunned me and took my breath away. The facts were there and could not be denied. I had been right from that first second when I rolled Stacy over on my living room floor. Regardless of how badly I wanted to be wrong—mistaken in that early diagnosis—my worst fear came true. In spite of the fact that I wanted to run away and not face it, the truth was there staring me in the face no matter where I turned. Stacy had suffered a stroke. In spite of my efforts to find an explanation—a cause for the hemorrhage in Stacy's brain—I found none. The damage was severe and permanent. Her life as we knew it had been irreversibly changed in an instant. We could not go back and undo it.

I could say we had no other choice but to accept what happened to Stacy but the truth is we *did*. It would have been easy to stand fixed, unmoving, hating the situation, and damning God, the world, and every person involved. We could have buried our heads, wallowed in self-pity, and allowed stroke to take everything—every last bit of us. We could have settled for what we were told could never be or we could thumb our noses and say, "We'll show you!"

We chose to take the road that led us through rougher terrain—the one that required a lot more effort than traveling the level path of least resistance.

On May 15, 2009, we gathered as a family to witness Camy and Dave exchange their marriage vows. Camy was an exquisite bride. At almost fifteen, Jordyn was stunning—so much like her mom was at her age. Little Ellie absolutely loved the entire day from start to finish. Patty, Jeannie, and Stacy stood together, holding hands—sisters joined in celebration. It was one of those special moments when we thanked God again for Stacy's survival. It showcased our family at its best.

The most poignant occasion in recent months was the passing of Stacy's former teacher, mentor and friend, Leah Griffin. Her battle with ALS came to an end on May 18, 2009. Stacy and I spent a few of her final quiet moments in the hospital room with her family. Leah's daughter Shari whispered in her mother's ear that Stacy was there. For a fleeting second Leah's almost non-existent breathing changed slightly. She knew Stacy was there to say goodbye.

Stacy was quiet—fighting back tears. She had not been able to see Leah for several weeks because of two rounds with a sinus infection that took a heavy toll on her energy level. She had emailed to arrange a visit but had not heard back. Now she knew why there had been no response. I waited, giving Stacy space to simply sit at Leah's bedside. After about an hour, she rose from her chair and came to say she wanted to leave. She needed to be away from the room and settle her own thoughts. It was simply too difficult for her to be so close to her own mortality.

Leah's memorial service was a touching celebration of life. Bouquets of flowers adorned the altar, but the pews were tied with brightly colored balloons—Leah's favorite. Stacy cried openly, resting her head on my shoulder, clasping my hand. What a remarkable woman Leah was. What a teacher. What a friend. What a loss.

One of Leah's favorite Bible passages was Ecclesiastes 3: 1-8. Stacy has spent time reading it again and again with new appreciation and has chosen it as one of her favorites as well. It reads,

> For everything there is a season, and a time for every purpose under heaven: a time to be born, and a time to die; a time to plant, and a time to pluck up that which is planted; a time to kill, and a time to heal; a time to break down, and a time to build up; a time to weep, and a time to laugh; a time to mourn, and a time to dance; a time to cast away stones, and a time to gather stones together; a time to embrace, and a time to refrain from embracing; a time to seek, and a time to lose; a time to keep, and a time to cast away; a time to tear, and a time to sew; a time to keep silence, and a time to speak; a time to love, and a time to hate; a time for war, and a time for peace.

The day after Leah's memorial service, Stacy came to my house wearing a bright yellow t-shirt that Leah had given her. On the front was a screen print of a sketch Leah made of an elephant she had met and came to love during her travels to Africa in the early 1970s. Stacy reminded me that the day would have been Leah's 67th birthday. She carried a note that Leah had written two years before when she was still able to hold a pen.

Dear Stacy—

> *I am so proud of you and so in awe of your strength and courage! Your paintings truly reflect your heart. Smile.*

Love, Leah

Chapter Twenty-Four

Postcards

*Faith consists of believing when it is beyond the power
of reason to believe.*

~Voltaire~

When I decided to write this book, the title came from our experience, from the name of Stacy's first collection of paintings, and also from the age-old idea that women are supposed to have the purgative to change their minds and give you a piece of them as they see fit. I raised my daughters to be independent thinkers and to stand up for themselves. *A Piece of Her Mind* seemed the rightful title for the story of what we've all been through.

It is impossible to thank every person who was instrumental in saving Stacy's life but whomever they are and wherever they may be, we are thankful for every one. We thank God that he gave the doctors the knowledge and expertise necessary to literally hold Stacy's brain in their hands and perform the delicate procedures that kept her alive. She is here with us today because of those individuals who did their duty guided by their life-saving oath. We believe God chose each of them very carefully.

Saving Stacy's life was only part of the plan. We know how blessed we have been to work with the professionals who gave Stacy her life back. We are so grateful for the PT and OT staff in Cheyenne who got the ball rolling. To the staff at Craig Hospital—Jean Milholland, Jennifer Quinn, and Lisa Strahn in particular—we owe a debt that has no price tag because it cannot possibly be repaid. They took Stacy's mind and body in their hands and taught it how to function again. They call themselves therapists but they are magicians!

We are also thankful for Bridget Scholljegerdes, Stacy's PT in Laramie, who picked up the therapy ball and ran with it. She never treated Stacy as if she was disabled but saw her as someone who could overcome the challenges in her path. Frances Price, Stacy's psychologist, is to be commended for helping heal her shattered soul. We are so grateful to Lynda Coyle for her endless hours of speech therapy and for falling in love with Stacy's art and her potential as an artist. Chris Primus and Athena Kennedy, Stacy's disability support team, went above and beyond the call of duty during Stacy's last semester of college. They share her degree because they never allowed her give up.

Make no mistake—we would never have reached the end of our journey without the support of our friends and family. We owe a huge thank-you to Tim and Mary Kingston, my cousin and her husband, who opened their home in Cheyenne to all of us. They are remarkably caring human beings who share whatever they have with whomever needs it.

I work with the best group of faculty and staff at the University of Wyoming. They are my co-workers and friends, and I appreciate each and every one of them. Special thanks to Suzy Pelican for reading through excerpts of my manuscript that I needed help with. We also adore our "partners in stroke" Larry and Vera Held and thank them for sharing with us as only stroke survivors can.

My siblings and our parents hold me and my children in their hearts and prayers every day. We are a wild and crazy bunch sometimes but we are just ordinary people who genuinely enjoy the lives God has blessed us with. My brother Arlin helped me put this special gift into perspective:

> Every single day since the day we were born, our parents have talked about us with the Creator of the universe. How awesome is that? *He* knows *us* by name. Our problems—trials and tribulations—have been laid at *His* feet. When our parents pray for their family, they include 85 people! That's every daughter, son, spouse, grandchild, great-grandchild, and so on. Mom and Dad humbly ask that we be given the strength, wisdom, and courage to meet whatever challenges come our way. Whenever we are hurt, sick, or troubled they pray without ceasing. That's the key. They have given us the greatest gift anyone could ever have. We have a pretty darn good family led by two amazing parents with an unwavering faith in God. Who could ask for anything more?

I asked the special people who joined Stacy and me on this journey if they would consider writing about what this experience has meant to them. I share their contributions with you now.

~

Stacy's sisters—her siblings, supporters, and friends—wrote messages from their hearts. The bond between my daughters has never waivered. It is stronger now than ever before. These women—my little girls—have grown into people I respect and admire. I am humbled by their strength. I love them more as each day passes.

From Camy:

When Mom asked me to put together something for her book, I wasn't sure what I wanted to say. We are a very animated family and I wasn't sure if my stories would work for all people who might read this.

When we were kids, Stacy was always the one to bring in the first dead thing she found. She always kept the neighbors on guard because she played army or cowboys and Indians. It's a wonder she didn't give someone a heart attack or a stroke!

As she got a little older she traded in her cap guns for paint brushes and has produced beautiful work both before and after her stoke. That is probably the one constant thing that she has had though out all of this.

When Stacy had her stoke she seemed so small—like a baby you wanted to protect and keep safe. For me the hardest part was watching her have to learn everything all over again. I think I took for granted all of the things I do everyday like going to work, eating by myself, and just being able to get out of bed.

In spite of all Stacy has had to go through, I am so proud of all the things she has accomplished. Literally having to learn how to eat and go to the bathroom by herself, she has come through it all with flying colors. It has been a long hard road for her and will be that way for the rest of her life. I hope that families who have to go through the same kind of situation we have will learn from our story.

From Patty:

When I went to visit Stacy that July while she was still at Craig Hospital, I attended her therapy sessions with her and was thrilled to see her moving more and talking more. I painted her toe nails and even witnessed some of her first steps with a walker. I cried! It was so touching to be there and see her slowly move her feet down the hall. Leaving that time wasn't much easier than in April when she was still so fragile. I knew the road ahead of her was long and bumpy, but she had already made more progress than many thought possible. This is the same fighting spirit of all the women in our family. We are tough and Stacy just kept on getting tougher and tougher.

Since that summer, Stacy has continuously amazed me. She never let a semester of college get the best of her. She worked really hard to get her driver's license, and when she was ready, she got her own place. As I came home to visit for Christmas breaks and summer vacations, I kept seeing this miracle in front of me. Her artwork reflected the pain and misery she went through, and when the time was right, she began to paint more and more.

She continued to plug away at school. Another amazing moment in her life since the stroke happened in December 2008—graduation from the University of Wyoming. I cried before the ceremony even started. My daughter Ellie ran out into the aisle when the procession began and yelled "Stacy!" Stacy stopped and bent down to hug her. The flood gates opened. I cried through the whole ceremony—the hardest when she walked across that stage. I kept thinking back to the day at Craig Hospital, when I saw those first few steps. Here she was without a cane or walker, just walking across the stage filled with pride.

I still stop and wonder why the stroke happened to Stacy. Was it to teach all of us something? Was to increase the intensity and message of her art? Was it some random medical fluke? What I do know is that it was no mistake on that late night in April 2003 when we agreed to fight for her life. The fighter inside Stacy has the same tenacity and phenomenal resilience I see in all of my sisters and our mom. Everyone who meets Stacy is immediately captivated by her heart, her love for life and her compassion for others.

In January 2009, Stacy began volunteering in my first grade classroom. She came once a week to help my students learn to illustrate their own stories. They were incredibly possessive of their "resident artist" and did not want to share her with their fellow first graders. Stacy surprised each of them with a sketch of their favorite animal. Not once did they notice or comment on any of her disabilities. When we had Disability Awareness Day at our school, I talked to my class about Stacy's stroke and her limitations. The ironic part about my attempt to educate them was that they argued with me and said, "No way—she does not!" I hope they remember that life lesson—they didn't see Stacy as different because they weren't looking for any differences—they just saw Stacy as an artist and a friend.

I am so proud of Stacy. She has been through more than any of us. On my worst day, I can't compare to the pain and suffering she endured. It makes sense that the rest of us have adopted her favorite saying—when you're going through hell, keep going!

From Jeannie:

I think I was in shock for several days. I walked around in a daze. When we walked into the hospital, Mom met us outside and warned us of what we were going to see. I was holding back tears as I walked into her room. She looked like she was just sleeping. Her cheeks were rosy and she really didn't look any different to me.

Throughout the time I was there, we all took turns staying with her around the clock, not only for her sake but for ours. I think we all gained comfort being there with her. She wasn't sleeping well. She would try to pull out her IV's and breathing tubes.

Sadly, I had to go back to Houston. I had to return to my job, my life. Leaving her was probably the most difficult thing I have ever had to do. She couldn't talk but she held my hand, crying, mouthing "NO!" as I was leaving. I felt an enormous amount of guilt for walking out of her room.

I had a very hard time coping. I was so far away and I always felt like I was out of the loop when it came to her progress. I was always thinking of her but I did not want anyone to pity me or her for what she had just gone through. I refused to use Stacy as a way for people to feel sorry for me so I stopped talking about it to my friends and kept all of my feelings to myself. I dove into my work and I probably distanced myself a little from her and my family.

I cried the first time I heard her voice on the phone. I didn't want her to know because I was afraid that it would make her upset. The one thing that has always stayed with me is that throughout this ordeal, she met every challenge and had a sense of humor about it. At one point, her head was swollen and she would joke that she looked like Sloth from the movie "Goonies". She would even joke and say the quote from the movie "Hey you guys!" I could tell that she was actually very self conscious and worried but she would never let anyone know that. She was always making everyone laugh.

What I appreciate about Stacy and the one thing that has never changed is the bond between Stacy and myself. We are only eighteen months apart in age and we shared a room as far back as I can remember. Stacy and I were almost polar opposites as kids. She was the tomboy where I was more of a girly-girl. We used to play together for hours though, whether it was with my Barbie dolls or her G.I. Joes. We always had so much fun together!

At one point she wore her hair very short and people thought I had a little brother. By the time Stacy got to high school, it was obvious that she was very much a girl. I remember her going to prom and people being shocked at how beautiful she was and that she "had legs". I guess you can't tell that when you wear jeans all of the time!

We never really fought as kids or even teenagers. I was always a little bigger than her and I used to sit on her chest. I wouldn't let her get up unless she said "You are the almighty Jeannie. I bow down to you." Of course, I only did that when Mom wasn't around.

Stacy has always been so creative and has been able to channel her artistic talents into so many areas. She is always "making" something. When I talk to her, I always ask what project she is working on. She is so selfless. Nearly everything she makes is for someone else.

She has continued to take her life in stride. I am so proud of everything she has accomplished. To think that a few years ago, a doctor told us that we would never have "our" Stacy back, that she might never walk or talk again. Now she has graduated from college, drives a car, and has her own place. What the doctors never knew was that "our" Stacy is one tough girl and we never would have lost her. She has grown into the most amazing person and has never lost her fighting spirit. Besides, she grew up having to put up with three older sisters and sharing one bathroom. Now that's a challenge!

~

My sister Myla is one of those people who could grow a garden in the middle of the desert or on top of the rockiest mountaintop. Her talent for growing things goes way beyond just having a green thumb. She embraces life, looks for beauty in everything she does, and thanks God every step of the way. She and I share that "female grizzly" designation I wrote about earlier. She has been my listening post more times than I can count. I never have to hold back when I unload on her. I love her dearly. She wrote these words:

When I first heard of Stacy's stroke, I immediately wanted to go to Mona's side and be of any help that I could, but having children of my own meant that was impossible. I instead went into "prayer warrior" mode. I asked the Lord to please take Stacy if there wasn't going to be any quality of life, but if she were to live to please give her the will to fight for whatever she would be able to recover . . . physically, mentally, and emotionally. I asked for strength beyond strength as we know it for Mona because I knew she was going to need it for a long time. I am amazed at the determination of them both. They have put aside all the "why me" thoughts and carried on in spite of many obstacles and the ignorance of others. I believe God has a great purpose for Stacy and for Mona, and has been revealing it all along. I am so proud of them.

Being a mother requires that "strength beyond strength." We carry and bear children and teach them to talk and walk knowing full well they will soon talk back and stomp away in anger. We need the strength to carry them when they are little, and then carry them through all the things that happen during adolescence. We need the strength to stand up for them and then the greater strength to stand back and let them fail, probably the hardest thing of all. We pray for them when they are little, and meet their needs daily. We learn to pray diligently and fervently when they are grown and we no longer are there to make the decisions and meet their needs. I am amazed at how much closer I have become to my Lord as my children get older and I see my children the same way He sees all of us. It is an amazing journey. God is good!

~

Our friend Treva Blumenshine Votipka was there before, during, and after Stacy's stroke. When we were in Cheyenne, she came to the hospital everyday on her lunch hour. She made us laugh, shared our tears, and encouraged us to keep going when we didn't think we could. We value her friendship and marvel at her faith. She sent the following:

A miracle is not something a person witnesses everyday, but I know that I have. From the first time I saw Stacy in ICU, my heart was confused. This outgoing, active, young lady now had tubes running all over her body. It just didn't seem right. I questioned why this was happening to her and her loving family. As time progressed the power of prayer and God's miracles were very obvious. Stacy has overcome so much and has been such an amazing inspiration to so many. I am very, very blessed to know Stacy and witness the miracle that she is.

~

My sister Callie and her family open their home to all members of our family who travel to Sheridan, Wyoming for various get-togethers. She never ceases to amaze me. She sees the good in everyone. She can pull a family event together in about five minutes and you'd think it took months. We love you, Callie, and want you to know how much we appreciate your thoughtfulness and generosity. She contributed this touching note:

My most vivid memory of Stacy is when she was probably 4 years old. She had broken her arm and had to stay in the hospital. Her mom had to go back home with the other girls so Stacy had to be alone for awhile. I remember going to see her. She looked so scared and she tried to be so brave. Her little chin just shook but she kept it together when we hugged her goodbye. It should have been an indication then of how strong she was going to be and that nothing was going to keep her down.

Our family has the ability to pull together whether we are miles away or right next to the hospital bed. The women in our family have endured many life challenges. We would not be who we are today without a strong maternal power to keep us going strong through all the trials. Our mother passed it on to us as mothers and us to our daughters and so on and so on. We are a powerful force to be reckoned with.

I didn't get to see Stacy in the hospital after her stroke but our mom, Grandma Dorothy, told us all the stories. I know that our mom's prayers work miracles. She can pray anyone through almost anything. She has proven that prayer is an amazing power.

Mona and her girls have been an inspiration to all women in this world. However we start in our lives, we can overcome adversity to be strong, independent, and powerful. Stacy had no choice but to follow the path of not letting anything stand in her way. From a tiny, little girl who was scared to this brave, strong, beautiful person she is today.

Stacy, you are an inspiration and miracle. Your life has been given back to you so you have a chance to be who you were meant to be. I can't wait to see all that you accomplish in your life. We can all learn from your perseverance and strength.

~

My friend and co-worker Tracy Bennett stepped in for me when I had to leave my job to care for Stacy. Her selfless gift of friendship is very precious to me. Thank you Tracy—for being you—a dear person, a hard worker, and a magnificent woman. She wrote:

The first time I met Stacy she was a spunky, ornery, funny high school girl. When I went to see her in the ICU after her stroke I could still see that spunk even with all the tubes running in and out of her mouth, nose, and arms; that is until she had a choking/coughing attack. Right after her stroke Stacy couldn't talk. It was hard for her to swallow, let alone cough. I don't know if I've ever been that scared for someone's life as I was at that moment. It still brings tears to my eyes thinking about it. As the nurses were flying around the ICU room trying to help Stacy, I noticed Mona stayed calm and strong. I knew with those family genes, Stacy would give it her all to get through the tough times ahead.

The next couple of hospital visits I saw the funny, ornery, and always spunky Stacy slowly coming back. Mona was always strong and determined. I'm not sure how she did it. I would have been a basket case if it were my child. Mona took care of Stacy and her job simultaneously without missing a beat. She was amazing in her own right. I believe Stacy gave Mona strength as Mona gave Stacy strength. After all the hard, hard work and pain Stacy has gone through the spunky, ornery, funny Stacy is still here with us today, and we are very blessed to have her. I have learned so much from both of these women—their strength and determination. My admiration for both is great. Thank you both for never giving up.

~

The following comes from Gena, my sister-in-law and cherished friend, who sat with us, prayed with us, laughed and cried with us. I will never be able to thank her enough for giving so much of herself to us. She is a remarkable woman and we love her very much. Thank you, Gena for your contribution.

After we got the call and Mom and I were headed to Cheyenne, we were just in shock. That a girl Stacy's age could have a stroke was just unheard of. I remember praying a lot and knowing that God was with us all. It was so hard seeing her laying in intensive care—so helpless. I also felt so helpless. I just wanted to fix everything. Knowing I couldn't was so hard. I knew that God had sent me there to be a support for you, Mona—to hold you, to cry with you, to pray with you, and to let you know that I was there for you no matter what. When we got the call from the hospital the night that you had to decide whether or not to operate was so hard. I can honestly say I would never want to be in that position. Then when the decision was made, we all just wanted to help.

I remember staying with Stacy a few nights and parts of some days. I knew I had to protect her. There was one time when the nurses came in to tend to her needs and they were rough with her. They didn't notice me sitting in the corner. I don't remember what I said but their attitude changed rather quickly. I wanted to just hit them. Wow, did I say that? The next day when they came in, they asked me to leave so I asked Stacy if she wanted me to stay. She nodded yes. So then I never wanted to see her left alone again. In my mind, I felt they thought that somehow this was Stacy's fault. I hated that.

Then I had to go home. Oh, how I hated to leave. I realized that there was nothing I could do. I felt so helpless. I am so glad that Stacy is here with us today. How I have enjoyed her. This has brought us—the whole family—and especially Stacy and you—closer than ever. That has been a blessing to me. I love you both so much. It was a privilege to be part of that time even though it was very hard. Stacy always makes me laugh. What a special woman she is.

~

My sister Wyonda has been my best friend for our entire lives. We have shared everything two sisters can. We are separated now by the distance between our homes but are only a thought and phone call apart. What I love most about her is the way she sees the world. She lives a simple life and never asks for anything other than what she has. I love her for always being there for me, for holding me up, for letting me cry and vent, and for sharing her special thoughts with Stacy and me. Her tender words of love follow:

When you hear the word stroke—you don't associate it with a vibrant, beautiful, healthy young girl. At first I was just so shocked. Stacy didn't drink, smoke or do drugs—no risk factors for stroke. She was just going to college and planning her future.

The night she lay near death will forever be etched in my mind. I lay awake all night—knowing in my heart that something had changed forever. I could feel all those thoughts and prayers going her way. She needed all of our strength if she was going to make it through. She was never far from our thoughts—the prayers were always coming.

One day when I was thinking about Stacy, I started singing the old hymn 'Stand by Me.'

> *When the storms of life are raging*
> *Stand by me*
> *When the storms of life are raging*
> *Stand by me*

When the world is tossing me
Like a ship out on the sea
Thou who rules wind and water
Stand by me

I knew Stacy couldn't sing it for herself—so I sang it for her—every day—several times a day—for months.

When I'm down and feel forgotten
Stand by me
When I'm down and feel forgotten
Stand by me
When I do the best I can
And nobody understands
Thou who never lost a battle
Stand by me.

To see Stacy now—what a miracle! She teaches me and others lessons every day. I want her to always know how special she really is—that she comes from a long line of incredibly tough women and that she can do anything. I wish her the very best.

~

My sister Loreen has been a strong mother figure to me for as long as I can remember. When I was little, Loreen was our second mom. She reminds me of stories I have read about some of the women in our family who lived and died long before we were born. Our family legacy of female strength definitely runs through her body. She wrote the following letter for Stacy and me. We love her very much.

No matter how much time passes, I will never forget Stacy's big eyes and bigger smile. She was a 'one of a kind' little girl. She had a savvy most kids don't have. She had to understand things far beyond her years.

No matter how much times passes; I will never forget the pain and fear in Stacy's eyes as I stood beside her hospital bed. The pain had awakened her. Her eyes pleaded with me for any help I could give her. All I could do was call a nurse. All the nurse could do was give more pain numbing medication. War had been declared.

There are moments, many moments, in all our lives when we feel hollow, like there is nothing left of us—no strength—no courage—not one ounce of being. But we stop—we wait—and we reach within to that reserve that our own mother silently gave to each of us and then we are ready to do battle.

I will never forget the look of complete despair on my sister's face in the hospital that day. There was fear in her eyes, in her voice, and in her hands as she reached for me to hold her close and try to lift a small piece of the burden that had been thrust upon her. My sister lost her 'little baby girl' that day. Stacy was grown, yes, but she had not yet become the woman she would have been. Stacy reached beyond all of that to become the woman she is today.

Stacy was born strong, but she had to become a fighter. She had to fight pain, prejudice, discrimination, bureaucracy, and disappointment. She had to learn that it is okay to be weak and to fail, and to do either does not mean you lose. I know Stacy fought hard to live even though at times she didn't even want to. The pain, fear, and confusion were more than overwhelming for her. Although Stacy suffered the stroke in her own brain, her heart was not the only one that suffered. Her life was not the only one changed forever.

Stacy had to find a courage that most of us know nothing about. And she did. She wears that courage not only as a medal, but as a crown and a royal cloak. And Stacy does not wear it alone—her mother stands wherever she needs to stand to do whatever she needs to do to help Stacy be whatever she can be.

Stacy honestly earns and deserves each and every commendation she receives—and her mother, for as long as she is able to do so, will be there to help her hold it.

~

Lacey is the youngest of the eleven children in our family. She occupies the same spot as Stacy—the baby of the family. We all love her and thank God daily for her renewed health. Her life too was hit by unexpected circumstances that shook us all to the depths of our souls. She knows what it's like to lean on your mom and sisters when you are too weak to stand alone. Her courageous battle with cancer was an experience at same level of fear and desperation that Stacy has endured. She shared her thoughts and her source of strength.

"Mommy, where's the eyes in the back of your head?" my six year old daughter asked as my husband shaved off what was left of my thick blonde hair. Being diagnosed with stage three breast cancer two weeks before my thirtieth birthday wasn't something I thought I would ever have to go through. Being the youngest of eleven children, I couldn't understand why God would want me to go through this.

Why not someone who was older? I had two small children and a lot of living left to do. I'd always had a relationship with God and Jesus and always felt that I was a good Christian, but what I wasn't doing was putting my whole trust in Him. This was something I couldn't run away from. He was going to be there with me all the way. "If God brings you to it . . . . He will bring you through it."

When Mona asked me to write a paragraph about "strength in the midst of tragedy," I thought about those days when I was so sick and the thought of dying and leaving my kids without a mom and my husband without a wife was so scary. But I always knew I wasn't alone at that time and even today. It is so hard to explain to someone who has never felt the presence of Jesus. He truly is your best friend at all times. God has given us all that incredible strength to get through those tough times, but the true test is the journey after the tragedy—the memories of the hard times and knowing that you can't just forget about them. That is what makes us strong and lets us know that He is there for us always. You just have to trust him.

Whenever I am having a bad day, I always think of our mother. I know that there must have been many times when she felt tired, lonely or completely stressed out. I know that her faith is what got her through. Even now as I look at her—she is not a big outspoken person—she is the strongest person I know.

In terms of Stacy, I think she has always been a unique individual. When I think of Stacy as she was before her stroke, and I look at her now, I have to say yes, she looks different, but Stacy is still Stacy. She speaks her mind, she has a great sense of humor, and I am amazed by this new independence that she has found. I don't think we are done seeing the great things that she will do, not only in her art but also in the way she influences others.

I asked Shayna, my own daughter, what she thought of the strong women in our family, but at thirteen she isn't quite sure how she feels about anything! As her mom, I can see her becoming another strong woman in our family. Shayna is a great leader and very much an individual. I know she will do great things in the future. The next generation is on its way!

~

My sister Loanna is one of the hardest working people I know. She takes care of everyone in her family and always goes above and beyond her job description as a wife and mother. She too has had her share of life's challenges. She takes them in stride and never lets them get her down. Our wish for her is that she have time to stop and enjoy the little things more often. She loves getting together with the entire family as often as she can. We appreciate her comments and love her very much.

I believe that if it wasn't for the love of her mother, continuous support of her big wonderful family, and a multitude of prayers, Stacy's life may have turned out differently. Never underestimate the power of prayer! Especially in this family!

~

My parents, Jack and Dorothy Cooper, are the most extraordinary people I know. I respect them, admire them, and love them more than I could ever put into words. Their faith has held our huge extended family together. Their approach to living—making the most of every single day—has been passed onto each of their children, grandchildren and so on. They welcomed Stacy for a week of vacation with them earlier this summer—her first without me since her stroke. She will always cherish that special time alone with her beloved grandparents—the two people who have prayed for her everyday of her life. They sent their special thoughts.

Dear Stacy:

When I think back over the years since that day we got the phone call telling us you were in intensive care in the hospital in Cheyenne and that you had had a stroke, I never cease to thank God for how far you have come and what a wonderful young lady you are today. To see you walk, drive your car, and travel alone is truly amazing! The road to where you are now has not been easy and you have known setbacks, but through it all you have had a great sense of humor and a desire to keep going.

May God bless you today and always,

Grandma Dorothy

Dear Stacy:

I think the fact that you have overcome almost insurmountable odds should be an example to many people, whether they are physically impaired or not. I admire your determination to never give up and though there are a few things you can't do, there are many things you can do. I am amazed at your self-reliance and of course, your sense of humor.

If only all people could know that there are going to be many rough spots in life—there are going to be mountains to climb, but remember, every mountain has a top and if that mountain was smooth, you couldn't climb it. May God bless you in all you do. May some of your dreams come true.

All the best,
Grandpa Jack

Chapter Twenty-Five

The Journey—In Her Own Words

I can be changed by what happens to me,
but I refuse to be reduced by it.

~Maya Angelou~

No one can tell this story better than Stacy herself. She has, from the very beginning, reached out with a willingness to share what happened to her and educate others. She could have handled this tragedy very differently—become bitter and disillusioned—but she has never pitied herself. I learn a new life lesson from her every day. She amazes me and I am so proud of her. She provides such astonishing insight into her stroke and recovery. Her words, strong and perceptive, provide our closing.

> *If someone asks me if I'm glad to be alive, I say, "Absolutely!"*
> *Am I grateful the doctors saved my life? Of course! Do I know how*
> *lucky I am to have my family beside me? Yes, I do. Do I wish this had*
> *never happened to me? I'd be lying if I said no. I am very thankful*
> *to be here but honestly, I miss the old me. I miss her everyday. I hate*
> *that I had a stroke and I wish it never happened.*
>
> *I cannot describe what it was like to be in the hospital bed*
> *looking at my arm. When Mom told me I was paralyzed I don't think*
> *it sunk in for awhile. I don't think it was that I didn't believe her.*
> *I think it was that I didn't want it to be true. I would lie in my bed*
> *trying to make my arm move. I tried to force it to move. I yelled at*
> *it. "Move, damn it! Move!" Then I begged. "Please move! Please.*
> *Move. Please!" But it never did.*

There were some really degrading times for me. No one should have to wear diapers when they are an adult. And having my mom wipe my butt because I couldn't was the worst! I couldn't dress myself or feed myself or take a bath or shower. I am glad I can take care of myself now.

I used to have dreams about running and doing everyday stuff. I still want to do the things I was able to do before my stroke. I hate the fact that my family can't so some things because I can't do those things anymore. Everyone has to walk slower when I'm with them because I can't walk as fast as they can.

I hate that I've gained weight and that I am not that cute skinny girl I used to be. I hate that I can't wear cute clothes and shoes. I wonder if I will ever meet a man who will love me like I am. I fear I will never have a chance at love. I want that very much.

Sometimes I get through the day without too much trouble. Other days I don't want to get out of bed. I am still hurt that my friends all turned away. I would never do that to someone and I can't understand why they did that to me. I have never gotten used to the way people stare at me. I am still Stacy on the inside and it hurts when people treat me like I'm retarded or something. I do not want people to feel sorry for me but I also don't want to be treated like I caused my stroke or that it was my fault somehow.

Some days I can't control my racing thoughts and I say whatever pops into my mind. Other times I struggle to find the right word or remember something that I read. It's weird how my brain works now. I fixate on something and I can't stop myself. My mom says I run without a filter. Some times I am obsessed with something I want to paint or build. It drives me nuts until I can make whatever I'm thinking about. I always have some sort of project going and I'm always asking my mom to help with it. I use her hands.

My art is my salvation. When I paint I don't have to think about my stroke. I painted before and I paint now. Stroke did not take that from me. Stroke does not define who I am.

I think every person has some kind of disability. Mine just happen to show on the outside. People who don't know how to love someone or how to appreciate the little things in life are way more disabled than I am. So are people who are mean or selfish or rude or discriminate against people like me.

I am not going to tell you my life is easy or that because I've been able to paint and finish college, I'm ok since my stroke. Yes, I survived my stroke but every day is a reminder of my old life. When I can't tie my shoes or any of those little things other people don't even think about, I get angry. In fact, it pisses me off that this happened to me. If there was any way I could go back in time and stop it from happening to me, I would. Stroke is ugly and awful and unfair. It destroys your life. It tried to kill me and it almost did but I fought back.

I hope you liked our book and will take something positive from my story. I want other people who have strokes or brain injuries to know they can still do things. I walk with a limp but I walk. I don't use a cane anymore. I use a leg brace sometimes when I hike with my family. I don't want to damage my million dollar leg! I have some movement in my left shoulder and elbow but none in my hand. I want to get that back so I keep trying to find ways to make that happen.

I have to ask for help sometimes and I hate when I have to do that. My mom and I have a rule—I have to try to do it by myself first and if I can't do it, she'll help me. Makes me crazy sometimes but usually I can do it by myself. She won't let me give up and I'm glad she doesn't. Stroke changed my life. It changed things for my family too. I appreciate them everyday for all they do with me and for me. I know I wouldn't be here without them and all they have done.

Will stroke ever stop me? No. Never. It tried. But I was stronger than stroke. I will always search for ways to do the things I want to do. I will never give up. I will never give in to my stroke.

I have a small magnet on my refrigerator. Mom put it in my Christmas stocking one year. It has the following quote by Erma Bombeck—a lesson we all should live by:

"When I stand before God at the end of my life, I would hope that I would not have a single bit of talent left, and could say, 'I used everything you gave me.' "